ISBN 978-0-9969501-4-5

Published by OnlineMedEd, www.onlinemeded.org
Authored by Dustyn Williams
Produced by Staci Weber

Reviewed and edited by John Andrew, Ryan Colakovic,
Dominique Cross, Dallin Elmer, Nathaniel Foster, Ran Jing, Austin Mahaffey,
Kiara Phelps, Nena Saini, Robert Shebiro, Thomas Stovall, Mateusz Tkacz

Printed in the United States of America

Congratulations on making it this far; the journey only gets harder from here. But you've found OnlineMedEd, and I'm here as your host for the next 1–6 years (depending on when you find me) to make your life a little easier. This book is part of that. You might be wondering, "what is this book Dr. Williams?"

- **It is:** A companion to OnlineMedEd's free Basic Sciences video lessons and a great place to take notes and reference our final whiteboards.

- **It isn't:** A shortcut or an excuse to skip writing out your own notes as you follow along.

As with everything we do, this book comes from OnlineMedEd's two steadfast principles:

- **Medical knowledge belongs to no one**, and so it is accessible to everyone. This is why the videos these whiteboards accompany are free and always will be.

- **OME's PACE learning methodology**—reading the notes (and taking your own), watching the video (and taking more notes), doing the challenge questions (and… wait for it… taking more notes), and enforcing it all through repetition—works. Purposeful engagement of the content in multiple modalities is the path to success.

This book is NOT a replacement for PACE. I've seen my students try to shortcut, and that's just not possible (or desirable) at the level you're looking to reach. I actually advocated that we not create this book as it might encourage you to skip steps by not writing out your notes or by not following along with our video lessons. To be clear, skipping steps like this will compromise your learning.

But I was overruled by you. We realized students were spending precious time and hundreds of dollars to print out the whiteboard graphics anyway, often in poor quality formats. So I acquiesced.

I designed the lessons to flow a certain way. To get the most out of them, follow PACE and follow along with my lessons at the board. The positioning on the board, the order in which the material is presented, the colors used, and even the cadences of speech are not accidental. It's all designed to help you understand what you need to understand when you need to understand it.

This book is a companion. It's not a crutch.

It also has a cute cat animation in the lower-left corner. Check it out.

Dustyn Williams, MD

Table of Contents

INFLAMMATION AND NEOPLASIA

IMMUNE

IMMUNOLOGY

MICROBIOLOGY

Genetic Material and Introduction OnlineMedEd

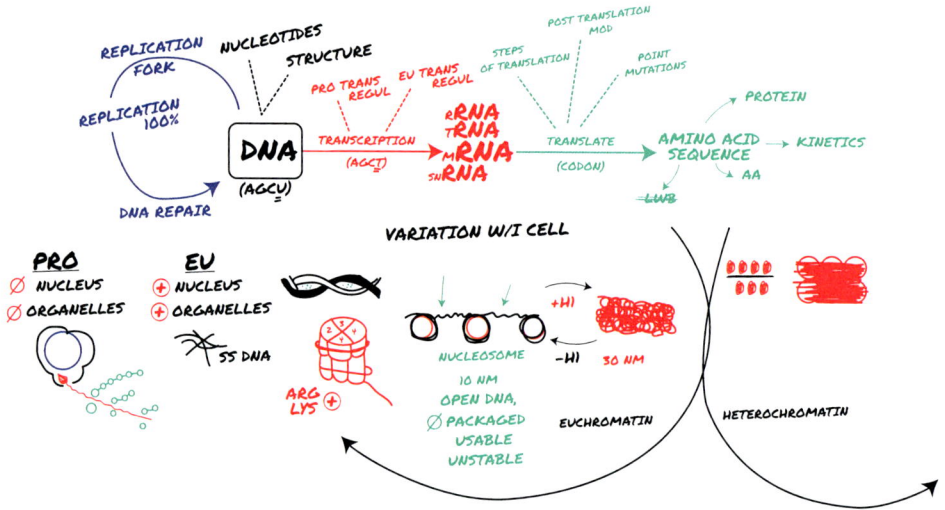

Nucleic Acids

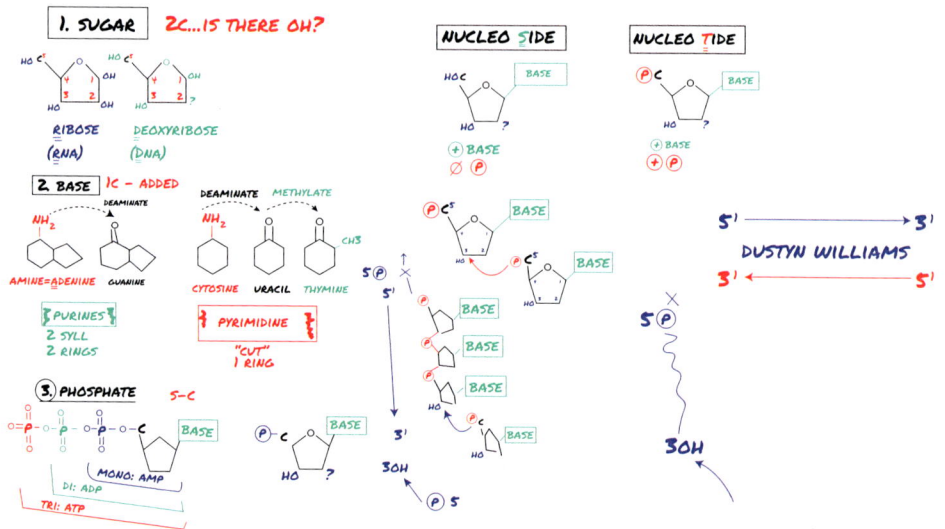

Structure of DNA

OH

5' · P · 5'

BASE T ÷ A BASE
BASE C ÷ G BASE
BASE G ÷ C BASE
BASE A ÷ T BASE

3'

CHARGAFF'S TOTALS
15% A = 15% T (30%)
35% G = 35% C (70%)

10,000
1000 A = 1000 T (2000) — 1000 A = T × 2 = 2000
4000 G = 4000 C (8000) — 4000 G ≡ C × 3 = 12000
14000

HYDROGEN BOND = 2E
G ≡ C
A ÷ T → 28,000

3'
HO

G ≡ C
A ÷ T
↑
WEAK

5'

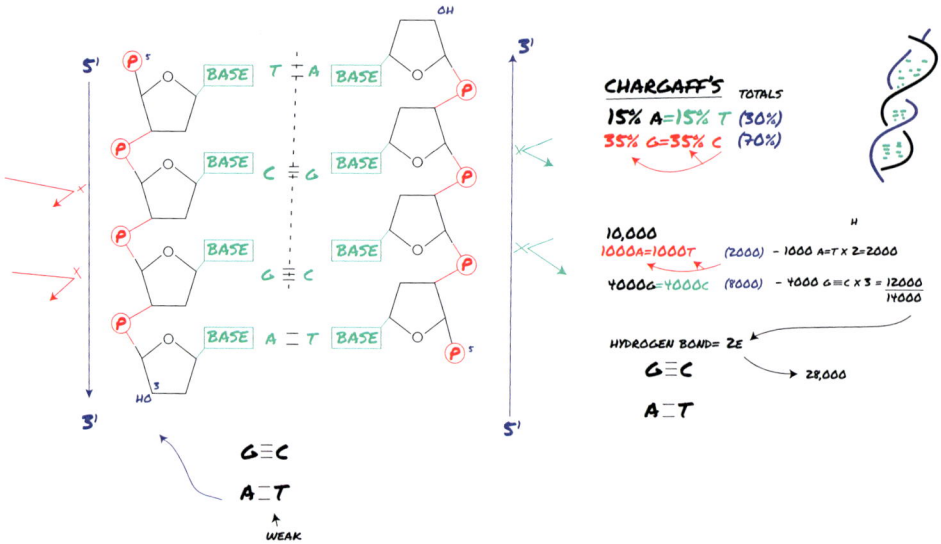

Intro to DNA and RNA

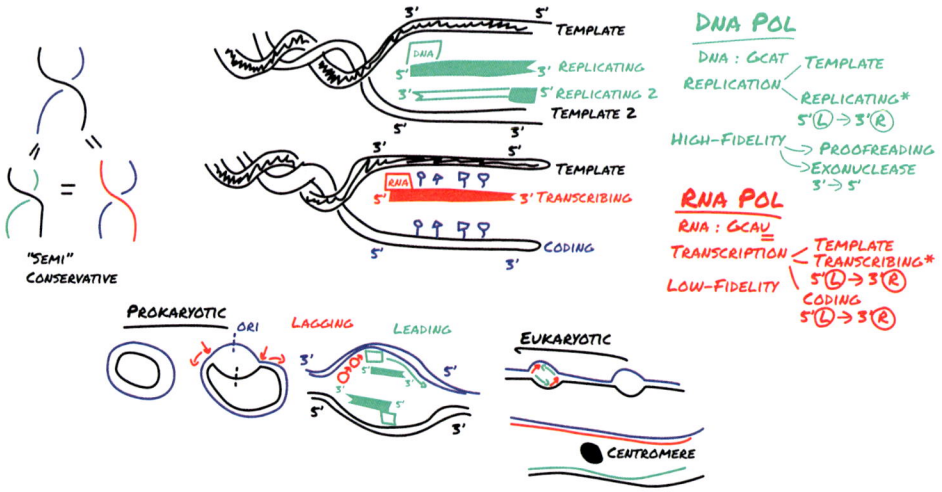

"SEMI" CONSERVATIVE

3' · · · · · 5' TEMPLATE
DNA
5' 3' REPLICATING
3' 5' REPLICATING 2
TEMPLATE 2
5' 3'

3' · · · · · 5' TEMPLATE
RNA
5' 3' TRANSCRIBING
CODING
5' 3'

DNA POL
DNA : GCAT TEMPLATE
REPLICATION REPLICATING*
5' (L) → 3' (R)
HIGH-FIDELITY → PROOFREADING
→ EXONUCLEASE
3' → 5'

RNA POL
RNA : GCAU
TRANSCRIPTION TEMPLATE
TRANSCRIBING*
LOW-FIDELITY 5' (L) → 3' (R)
CODING
5' (L) → 3' (R)

PROKARYOTIC
ORI
LAGGING LEADING
3' 5'
5' 3'
5' 3'
5' 3'

EUKARYOTIC

CENTROMERE

10

© 2020 OnlineMedEd

DNA Replication (The Fork)

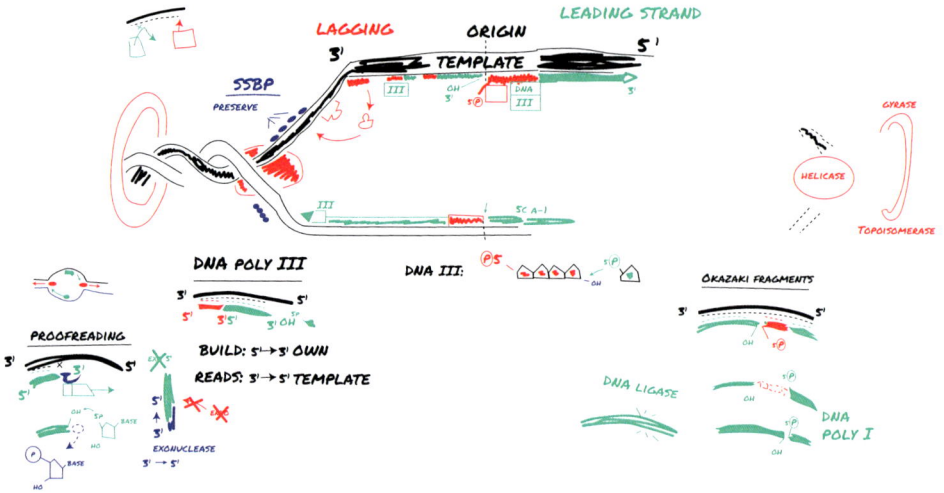

DNA Synthesis Repair

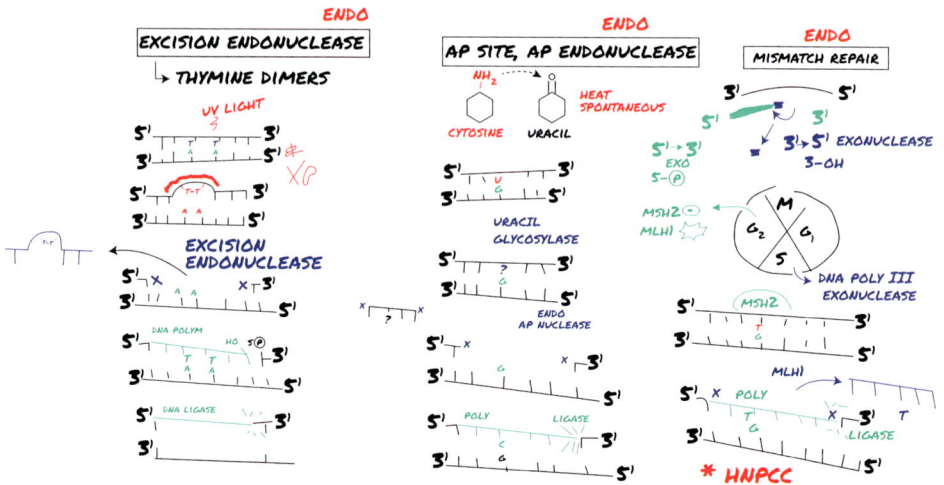

Introduction to Transcription

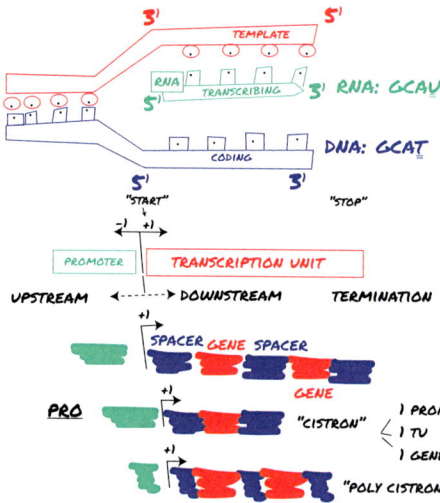

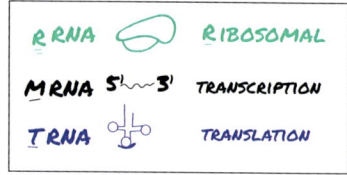

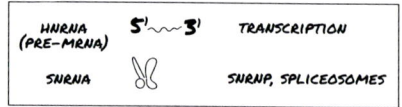

Prokaryotic Transcription

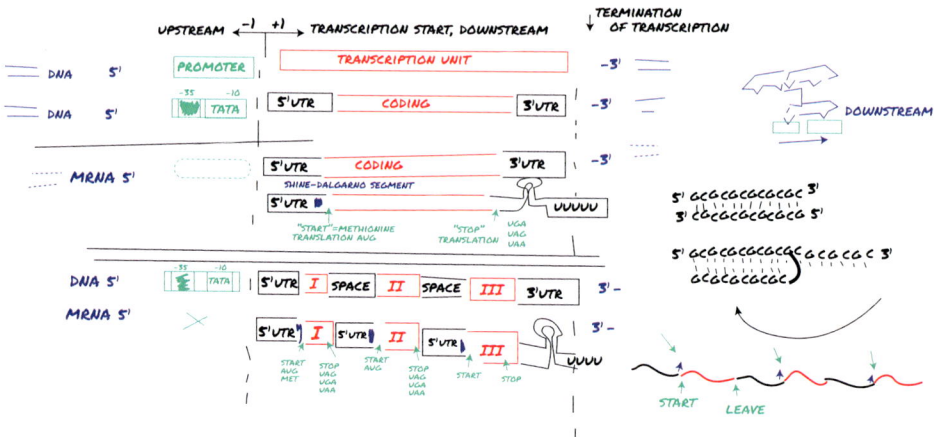

NOTES

Eukaryotic Transcription

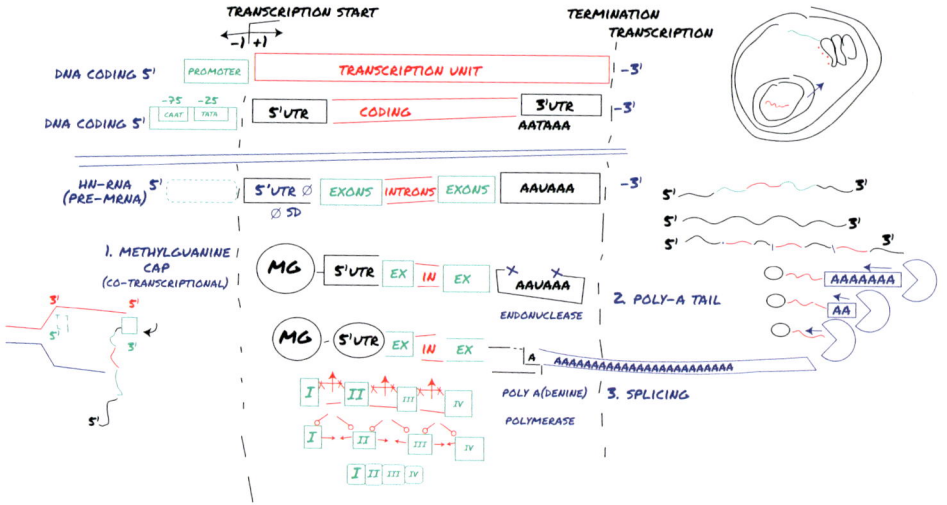

Eukaryotic Transcription Regulation

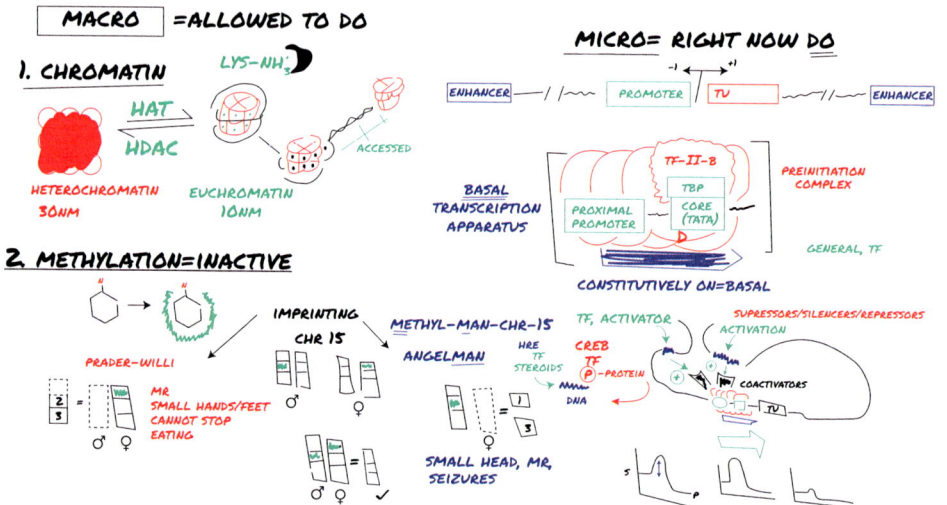

Prokaryotic Transcription Regulation

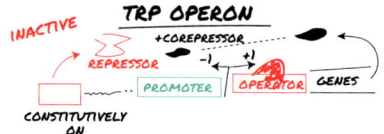

LAC OPERON

IF   ∅ GLUCOSE   ↓ ~~GLUCOSE~~   ↓ ATP   ↑ cAMP

AND   ⊕ LACTOSE   ↑LACTOSE=SEQUESTERS I-PROTEIN DISINHIBIT

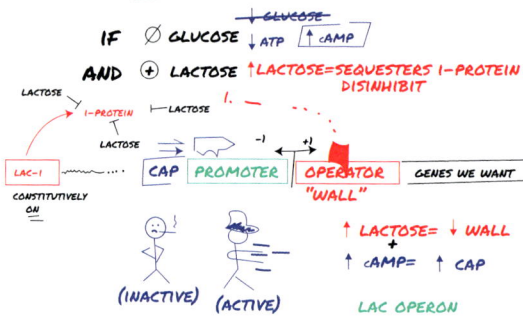

LACTOSE → I-PROTEIN — LACTOSE

LACTOSE

LAC-1 constitutively ON •••• ~~CAP~~ PROMOTER OPERATOR GENES WE WANT "WALL"

(INACTIVE)   (ACTIVE)

↑ LACTOSE= ↓ WALL
+
↑ cAMP= ↑ CAP

LAC OPERON

TRP OPERON

INACTIVE   +COREPRESSOR

REPRESSOR   -1   +1   PROMOTER   OPERATOR   GENES

constitutively ON

ATTENUATION

LEAD

– CODING 5' — I — II — III — IV — 3'–

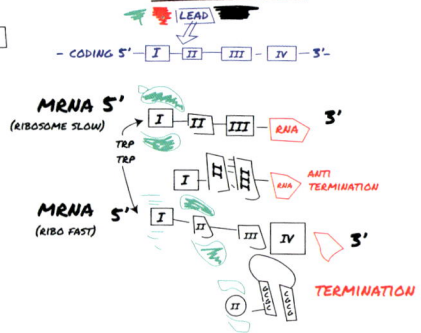

MRNA 5' (RIBOSOME SLOW)   I — II — III — RNA   3'
TRP TRP

I   II   III   RNA   ANTI TERMINATION

MRNA 5' (RIBO FAST)   I   II   III   IV   3'

II   TERMINATION

Intro to Translation

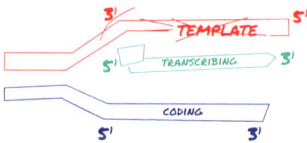
3' — TEMPLATE — 5'
5' — TRANSCRIBING — 3'
5' — CODING — 3'

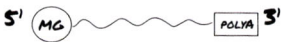

5' (MG) ~~~~ POLYA 3'

5' ~~~~ 3' MRNA

(N) NH₂–◯–◯–◯– COOH   +   NH₂ ◯– COOH (C)

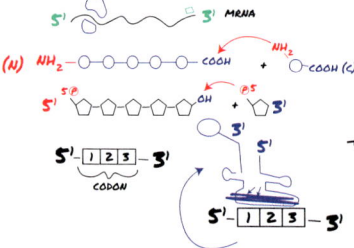

5' 1 2 3 3' CODON

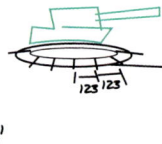
123 123

5' 1 2 3 3'

CODES + CODONS

1. UNIVERSAL
2. UNAMBIGUOUS   1–CODON=1–AA=1 TRNA
3. DEGENERATE   3 NT, 4BP
   (REDUNDANT)   64 CODONS
   ↳ "WOBBLY BP"   20 AMINO ACIDS
* 4. NONOVERLAPPING
   +
   COMMALESS   5'– 1 2 3 –3'
   NO GAPS, NO REUSED
   NO SKIPS.
5. "START" = AUG = MET
6. "STOP"= UGA
          UAG } ∅ AA
          UAA

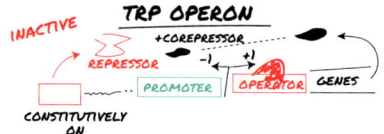

DNA to Protein

Translation

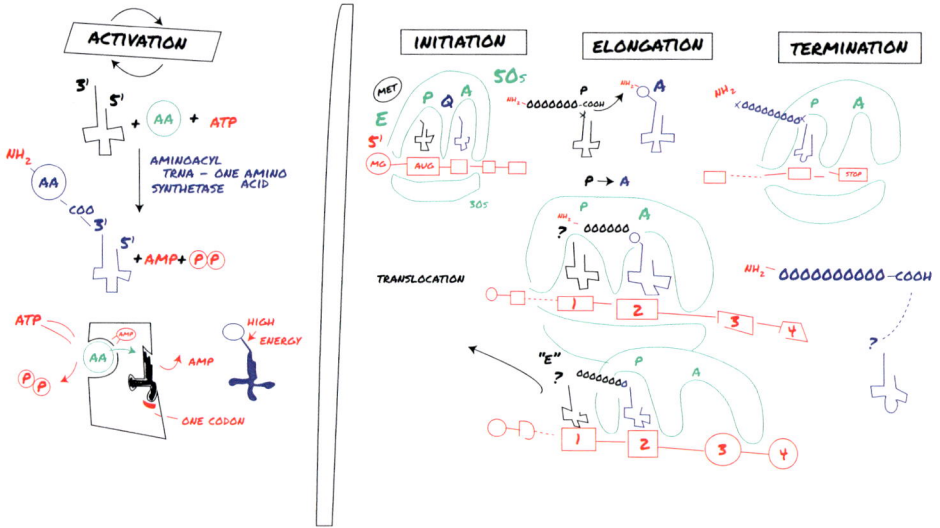

Post-Translational Modification

FOLDING + MISFOLDING

1°: AMINO ACID
LINEAR SEQUENCE

N-O-O-O-O---O-COOH

2°: 2D
β-SHEETS
α-HELIX

3°: 3D SHAPES

4°: SUBUNITS COMBINE

CHAPERONES
"✓"

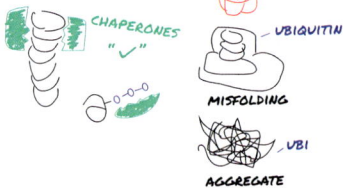

UBIQUITIN
UBI

MISFOLDING

AGGREGATE
UBI

PEPTIDE CLEAVAGE

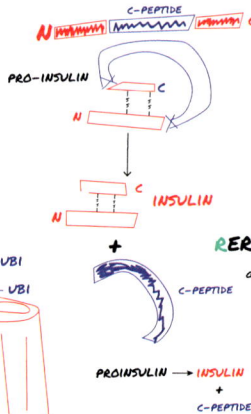

C-PEPTIDE
N C

PRO-INSULIN

C
N
INSULIN

+

UBI
UBI
UBI

RER
GOLGI

C-PEPTIDE

PROINSULIN → INSULIN
+
C-PEPTIDE

DESTINATION

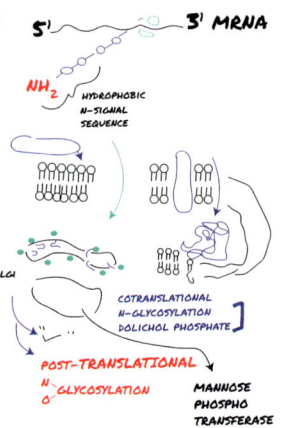

5' 3' MRNA

NH_2 HYDROPHOBIC
N-SIGNAL
SEQUENCE

COTRANSLATIONAL
N-GLYCOSYLATION
DOLICHOL PHOSPHATE

POST-TRANSLATIONAL
N-
O-GLYCOSYLATION

MANNOSE
PHOSPHO
TRANSFERASE

DNA to Protein

Point Mutations

POINT MUTATIONS = ONE NUCLEOTIDE

↳ TRANSITION (PUR->PUR, PYR->PYR)

↳ TRANSVERSION (PUR<->PYR)

SILENT
- ⊕ △ DNA
- ∅ △ PHENOTYPE
- ∅ △ AA SEQUENCE

64 CODONS
20 AMINO ACIDS
WOBBLY CODON
3RD POSITION

MISSENSE = MISTAKE
- ⊕ △ DNA
- ⊕ △ PHENOTYPE ... STILLWORKS
- ⊕ △ AA

HGBSS, AR
CHR 11
POS 6
GLU → VALINE
GAG   GUG

NONSENSE = NO SENSE
- ⊕ △ DNA
- ⊕ △ PHENOTYPE ✗〰
- ⊕ CATASTROPHIC

SHORTER

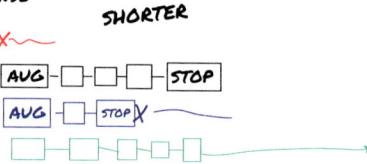

FRAMESHIFT MUTATIONS

LEU SER VAL THR
(UCAGCGUUACCU
SER ALA LEU PRO

NONSENSE

SPLICE SITE MUTATIONS

ADD SPLICE
REMOVE SPLICE

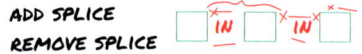

LONGER

Amino Acids

AMINO ACID

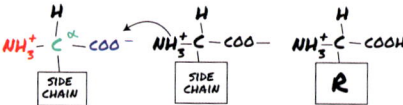

$NH_3^+ - C^\alpha - COO^-$ SIDE CHAIN

$NH_3^+ - C - COO^-$ SIDE CHAIN

$NH_3^+ - C - COOH$ R

PH AND PK

PH NH_3^+ 9
PK COOH 2

$NH_3^+ \rightleftharpoons NH_2 + H^+$
$COOH \rightleftharpoons COO^- + H^+$

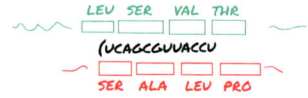

H+ H+ H+   PH=7.4

PK	SOL MORE ACID?	SOL MORE H+?	SOL WHAT DO?	NH COO-
NH_3: 9	MORE ACID	MORE H+	DONATE H+	NH_3^+
COOH: 2	LESS ACID	LESS H+	ACCEPT H+	COO-

ORGANIZATION OF AMINO ACIDS
★ = ESSENTIAL

HYDROPHOBIC (NOT CHARGED, NOT POLAR)

ALIPHATIC

GLYCINE GLY | ALANINE ALA | VALINE VAL ★ | LEUCINE LEU ★ | ISOLEUCINE ILE ★

AROMATIC

PHENYLALANINE PHE ★ | TYROSINE TYR | TRYPTOPHAN TRP ★

HYDROPHILIC (CHARGED OR POLAR)

"BASIC" + CHARGE
EXTRA NH_3^+ ~ NH_2^+, PKA=9

LYSINE LYS ★ | ARGININE ARG ★ | HISTIDINE HIS ★

"ACIDIC" — CHARGED
EXTRA COO ~ COOH, PKA=2

ASPARTIC ACID ASP | GLUTAMIC ACID GLU

—OH

SERINE SER | THREONINE THR ★

"NEUTRAL" POLAR, UN-CHARGED

SULFA

CYSTEINE CYS | METHIONINE MET ★

OTHER

GLUTAMINE GLN | ASPARAGINE ASN

GLYCOSYLATION

DNA to Protein

Enzyme Kinetics

$\triangle$G: IS THIS RXN SPONTANEOUS? (REVERSIBLE?)

$\triangle$G = GP-GS

$\triangle$G>0 ∅
$\triangle$G=0
$\triangle$G<0 SPONTANEOUS IRREVERSIBLE

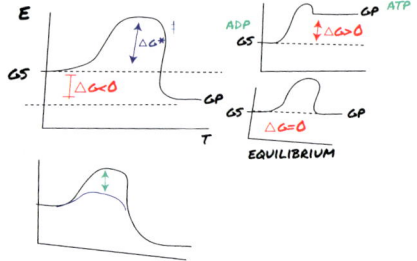

V RATE OF REACTION

VELOCITY
ACTIVATION
ENERGY

$\uparrow \triangle G^* = \downarrow$ RATE, $\downarrow$ V
$\downarrow \triangle G^* = \uparrow$ RATE, $\uparrow$ V

ENZYMES
$\downarrow \triangle G^*$
$\uparrow$ V

VELOCITY

$\uparrow$ UMAX
$\uparrow$ ENZYME

"SATURATED"

25%

KM KM

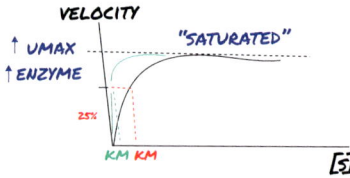

$[\underline{S}]$

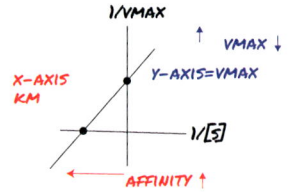

$\uparrow$ VMAX = $\uparrow$ #SITES

$\uparrow$ KM $\downarrow$ AFFINITY

1/VMAX

$\uparrow$ VMAX $\downarrow$
Y-AXIS=VMAX

X-AXIS
KM

$1/[\underline{S}]$

AFFINITY $\uparrow$

Inhibitors and Activators

1. $\uparrow$ Y-AXIS, $\downarrow$ VMAX

2. $\leftarrow$ X-AXIS, $\downarrow$ KM
$\uparrow$ AFFINITY

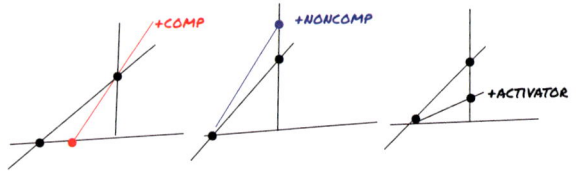

+COMP   +NONCOMP   +ACTIVATOR

3. COMPETITIVE INHIBITIONS — $\uparrow$ KM, AFFINITY$\downarrow$ $\longrightarrow$ X-AXIS — ∅ VMAX, ∅$\triangle$ Y-AXIS

4. NONCOMPETITIVE INHIBITIONS — ∅$\triangle$ KM, ∅$\triangle$ X-AXIS — $\downarrow$VMAX, $\uparrow$ Y-AXIS

5. ACTIVATORS "MORE ENZYME" — ∅$\triangle$ KM, ∅$\triangle$ X-AXIS — $\uparrow$VMAX, $\downarrow$ Y-AXIS

N O T E S

DNA to Protein

OnlineMedEd

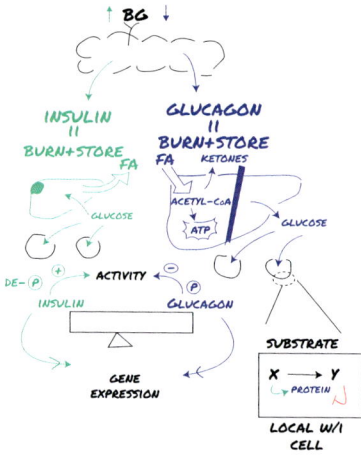

	Ø MITO	MITOCHONDRIA / DOWNTIME	DOWNTIME		
	RBC	BRAIN	SK MUS	ADIPOSE	LIVER
#3 GLYCOLYSIS	+	+	+	+	+
#4 PDH #5 TCA #6/#7 ETC	−	+	+	+	+
#8 GLUCONEOGENESIS	−	−	−	−	+
#9 REGULATION #10 FRU/GAL					
#11/#12 GLYCOGEN	−	−	+	+	+
#14/#13 FA SYNTHESIS	−	−	−	+	+
#15 FA OXIDATION	−	−	+	+	+
KETONES	−	+	+	+	MAKE
#17 SPHING					
#18-20 AA	−	−	+	−	+

PATHWAYS, REGULATION, ENERGY

Glycolysis

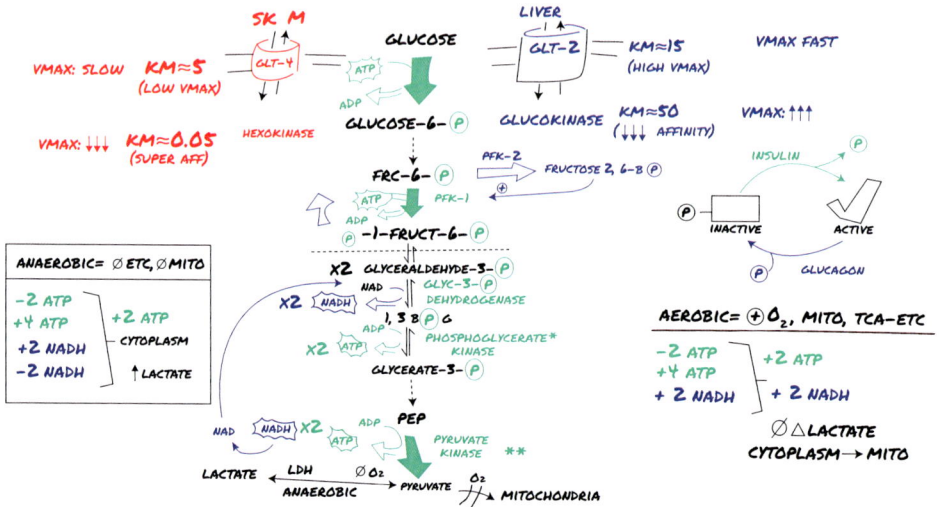

Metabolism

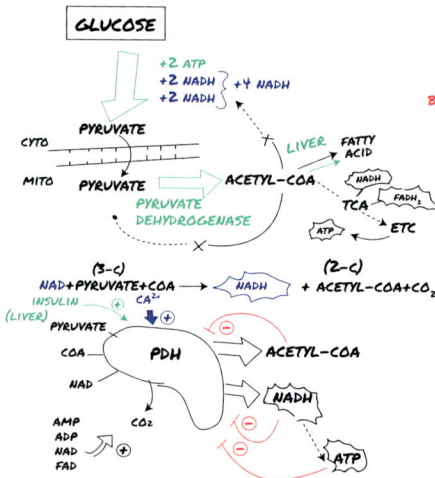

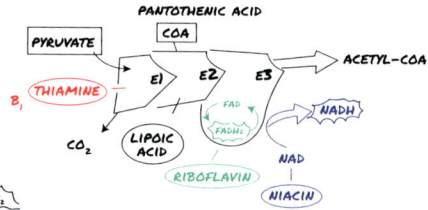

Pyruvate Dehydrogenase

GLUCOSE

+2 ATP
+2 NADH
+2 NADH } +4 NADH

PYRUVATE

CYTO

MITO   PYRUVATE

LIVER   FATTY ACID

PYRUVATE DEHYDROGENASE   ACETYL-COA

NADH
TCA   FADH₂
ATP   ETC

(3-C)
NAD+PYRUVATE+COA → NADH
INSULIN (LIVER)   Ca²⁺ +

(2-C)
+ ACETYL-COA+CO₂

PYRUVATE
COA
NAD
PDH   ACETYL-COA

AMP
ADP   CO₂
NAD
FAD   +   NADH
ATP

PANTOTHENIC ACID

PYRUVATE   COA   ACETYL-COA

B₁   THIAMINE   E1 E2 E3

CO₂   LIPOIC ACID   FAD
FADH₂   NADH

NAD
RIBOFLAVIN   NIACIN

THIAMINE DEF

ETOH ─┤   → THIAMINE   ∅ PDH= ∅ ACETYL-COA
∅ TCA=   ∅ ATP
= HFREF, "WET" BERI-BERI   ∅ AA CATAB

REVERSIBLE   IRREVERSIBLE   KETONES
=
W   K

ATAXIA
NYSTAGMUS   MEMORY LOSS   COMA
ENCEPHALOPATHY   CONFABULATION

COMA COCKTAIL

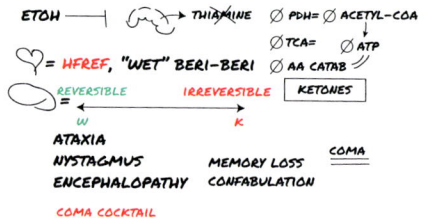

Citric Acid Cycle

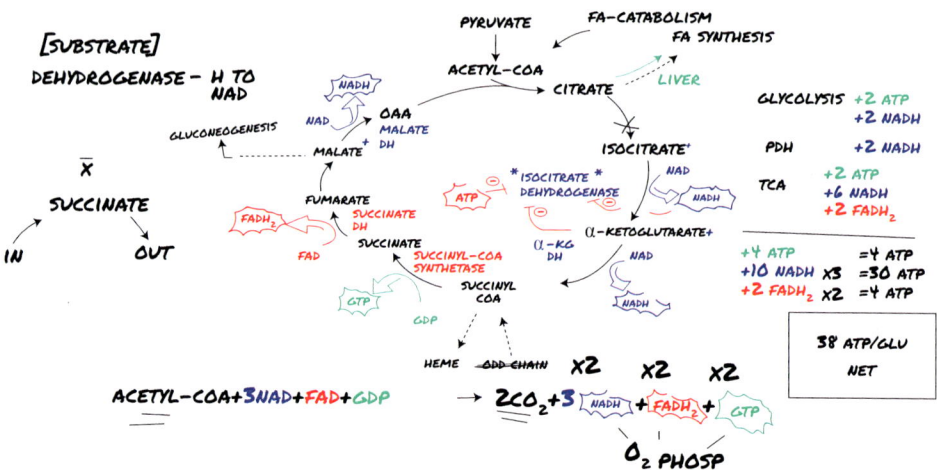

[SUBSTRATE]
DEHYDROGENASE - H TO NAD

PYRUVATE
ACETYL-COA   FA-CATABOLISM
FA SYNTHESIS

CITRATE   LIVER

GLUCONEOGENESIS
NADH
NAD   OAA   MALATE
MALATE   DH

X̄
FUMARATE   ISOCITRATE*

SUCCINATE   ATP   * ISOCITRATE *
DEHYDROGENASE   NAD

IN   OUT   FADH₂   SUCCINATE DH
FAD   SUCCINATE   α-KETOGLUTARATE+
SUCCINYL-COA   NADH
SYNTHETASE   α-KG
DH   NAD
GTP   SUCCINYL COA   NADH
GDP

GLYCOLYSIS +2 ATP
+2 NADH

PDH   +2 NADH

TCA   +2 ATP
+6 NADH
+2 FADH₂

+4 ATP   =4 ATP
+10 NADH ×3 =30 ATP
+2 FADH₂ ×2 =4 ATP

38 ATP/GLU
NET

HEME   ODD CHAIN   ×2   ×2   ×2
ACETYL-COA+3NAD+FAD+GDP   → 2CO₂+3 NADH + FADH₂ + GTP
O₂ PHOSP

Metabolism

Electron Transport Chain

SYNTHESIS **COST ENERGY**

NADH FADH$_2$ CYTO I Q II III IV O$_2$

GLUCOSE
+2 ATP
+2 NADH

✓LACTIC ACID: POOR TISSUE PERFUSION

~~LDH: INFLAMMATION~~ ATP → ADP

TROPONIN I:

CYTOPLASM ↑ LACTATE ←LDH← PYRUVATE

OUTER H+

MALATE 3ᵗʰ GLYC SHUTTLE

ATP ADP TRANSLOCASE

INTERMEMBRANE SPACE H+ H⁺ H⁺ H⁺

INNER H⁺ H⁺

MITOCHONDRIA I Q II FADH$_2$ FAD

CYT C

III (FE) IV (CU)

H⁺ H⁺ H⁺ H⁺ H⁺

FoF₁ ATP SYNTHASE

NADH 3ATP NAD 2 ATP

O$_2$

ATP

ADP

$\overline{X}$ RBC

NADH
PDH

NADH FADH$_2$ NADH
TCA FA CATABOLISM

38 NET/GLUCOSE= O$_2$
2 NET/GLUCOSE= ∅
5% ATP $\overline{5}$ O$_2$

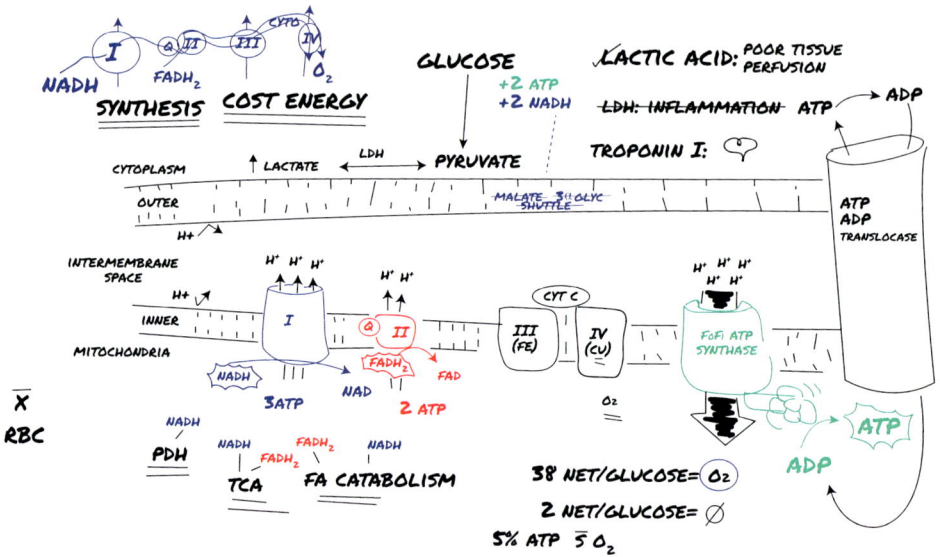

Electron Transport Pharmacology

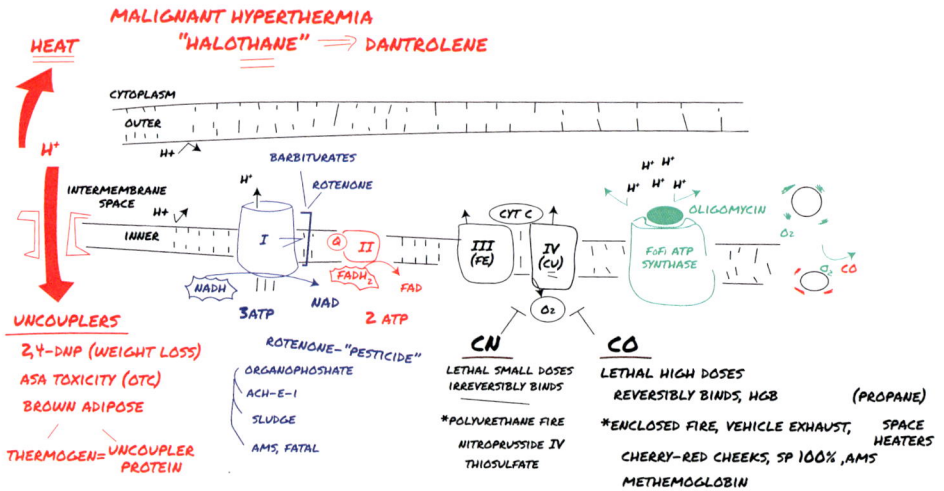

MALIGNANT HYPERTHERMIA
"HALOTHANE" ⟹ DANTROLENE

HEAT

H⁺

CYTOPLASM
OUTER H+
INTERMEMBRANE SPACE H+

BARBITURATES ROTENONE

INNER

I Q II FADH$_2$ FAD
NADH 3ATP NAD 2 ATP

CYT C
III (FE) IV (CU)

H⁺ H⁺
H⁺ H⁺ H⁺

OLIGOMYCIN

O$_2$

FoF₁ ATP SYNTHASE

O$_2$ CO

CN CO

UNCOUPLERS
2,4-DNP (WEIGHT LOSS)
ASA TOXICITY (OTC)
BROWN ADIPOSE

THERMOGEN= UNCOUPLER PROTEIN

ROTENONE- "PESTICIDE"
ORGANOPHOSHATE
ACH-E-I
SLUDGE
AMS, FATAL

CN
LETHAL SMALL DOSES
IRREVERSIBLY BINDS

*POLYURETHANE FIRE
NITROPRUSSIDE IV
THIOSULFATE

CO
LETHAL HIGH DOSES
REVERSIBLY BINDS, HGB (PROPANE)

*ENCLOSED FIRE, VEHICLE EXHAUST, SPACE HEATERS
CHERRY-RED CHEEKS, SP 100% ,AMS
METHEMOGLOBIN

Metabolism

Gluconeogenesis

KETONES **GLUCAGON-DOMINANT**

↓↓ * GLUCOKINASE   → INDUCES—INSULIN ↓↓

GLUCOSE → GLUCOSE-6-(P)

GLUCOSE → ↑↑ ATP? ↑↑

GLUCOSE-6-P PHOSPHATASE

GLUCOSE → ✕ → GLUCOSE

FA   ACETYL-COA

GLUCOSE

GLYCOGEN

FR-6-(P)   PFK-2 → FR-2,6-BP

(+) PFK-1 (−)   INSULIN

FR-1,6-BI PHOSPHATASE   (+)   (P) → PFK-2 → ACTIVE ✓

FR-1,6-BI (P)   INACTIVE

(P) → GLUCAGON (P)

SUBSTRATE: PDH (−)   (PEPCK) PEP CARBOXYKINASE

PC ← **ACETYL-COA** (+)

GLUCAGON INDUCES

PEP 3-C (+) P

OAA 4-C Ø (P)   PYRUVATE KINASES

(P) STATES: ↓ PDH   ↓ INSULIN   PYRUVATE   CYTO

↓↓ PFK-2   ↓ DE (P)   MALATE SHUTTLE   MITO

↓ INSULIN ↓ DEP   OAA   PYRUVATE   INSULIN ↓↓

↑ GLUCAGON ↑ (P)   4-C   PYRUVATE 3-C Ø (P)   PDH (−) ACETYL-COA ← FA

INDUCTION: ↓ GLUCOKINASE ↓ INSULIN   Ø (P)   CARBOXYLASE   OAA → CITRATE

↑ PEPCK   ↑ GLUCAGON   (+)   TCA ETC

Carbohydrate Regulation

INDUCTION HORMONE — (P) STATES   GLUCOSE   INSULIN   FA

(WHOLE-BODY)   GLUCOSE-6 PHOSPHATASE   GLUCOKINASE   INSULIN   GLUCOSE

INSULIN-DOM   GLUCAGON-DOM   GLUCOSE-6-(P)   KETONES   FA

GLYCOLYSIS   GLUCONEOGENESIS   INSULIN (+) GLUCAGON   GLUCAGON   GLUCOSE

(+) INSULIN   (−) INSULIN   FR-6-(P)   PFK-2 (+)(+)(−)

(+) GLUCAGON   (+) FBP   PFK-1   FR26   ↑INSULIN ↑PDH   ↓INSULIN ↓PDH

FR-1,6-BI (P)   ↑GLUCOKINASE   ↓GLUCOKINASE

SUBSTRATE = PRIORITY   GLUCAGON   ↑PFK-1 ↑PFK-2   ↓PFK-2 ↓PFK-1

(CELL-LEVEL)   PEPCK   ↑GLUCAGON ↑ PEPCK

OAA   PEP   ↑FBP ↓PFK-2

LOW   HIGH   MALATE   PYRUVATE KINASE   FA SYNTHESIS

AMP   ATP   PYRUVATE

ADP   OAA   ACETYL-COA ← FA CATABOLISM

NAD   NADH   PYRUVATE   PDH

FAD   FADH2   PYRUVATE CARBOXYLASE   TCA

ACETYL-COA   (+)   ETC → ATP

INSULIN

Metabolism

Galactose and Fructose

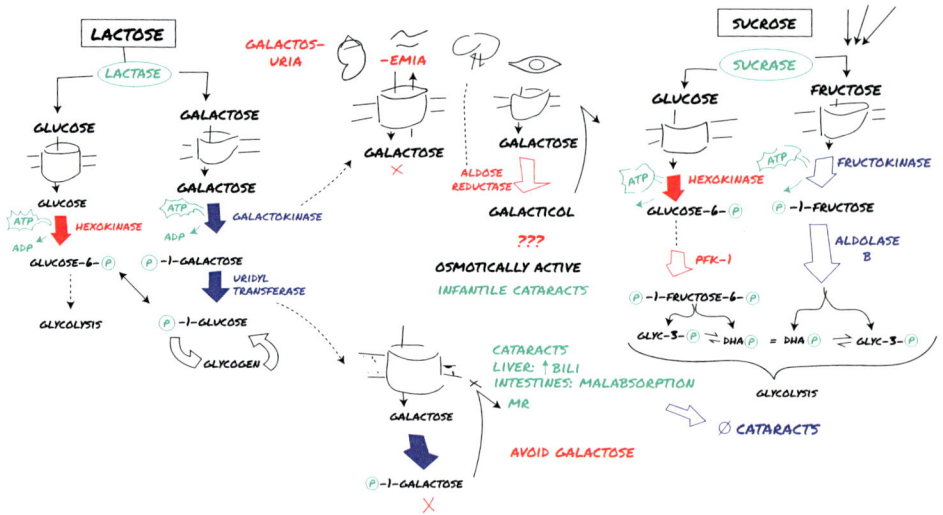

LACTOSE

LACTASE

GALACTOS-URIA — ─EMIA

GLUCOSE   GALACTOSE

GALACTOSE   GALACTOSE

GALACTOSE

GLUCOSE
ATP HEXOKINASE
ADP
GLUCOSE-6-Ⓟ

GALACTOSE ✕

ADP GALACTOKINASE
ATP
Ⓟ-1-GALACTOSE
URIDYL TRANSFERASE
Ⓟ-1-GLUCOSE

GLYCOLYSIS

GLYCOGEN

ALDOSE REDUCTASE
GALACTITOL
???
OSMOTICALLY ACTIVE
INFANTILE CATARACTS

GALACTOSE
Ⓟ-1-GALACTOSE ✕

CATARACTS
LIVER: ↑BILI
INTESTINES: MALABSORPTION
MR

AVOID GALACTOSE

SUCROSE

SUCRASE

GLUCOSE   FRUCTOSE

ATP HEXOKINASE   ATP FRUCTOKINASE
GLUCOSE-6-Ⓟ   Ⓟ-1-FRUCTOSE

PFK-1   ALDOLASE B

Ⓟ-1-FRUCTOSE-6-Ⓟ

GLYC-3-Ⓟ ⇄ DHA Ⓟ = DHA Ⓟ ⇄ GLYC-3-Ⓟ

GLYCOLYSIS

Ø CATARACTS

Glycogen Metabolism

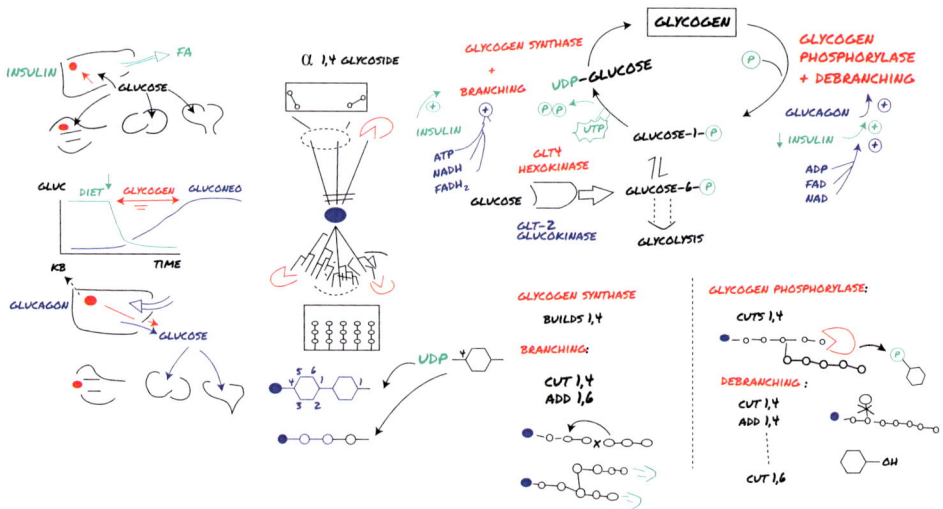

INSULIN   FA
GLUCOSE

GLUC DIET GLYCOGEN GLUCONEO
=
KB   TIME

GLUCAGON
GLUCOSE

α 1,4 GLYCOSIDE

UDP

GLYCOGEN

GLYCOGEN SYNTHASE
+
BRANCHING   UDP-GLUCOSE

INSULIN
ATP
NADH
FADH₂
GLUCOSE

GLT4
HEXOKINASE

GLT-2
GLUCOKINASE

Ⓟ Ⓟ
UTP
GLUCOSE-1-Ⓟ

GLUCOSE-6-Ⓟ

GLYCOLYSIS

Ⓟ

GLYCOGEN PHOSPHORYLASE + DEBRANCHING

GLUCAGON   +
↓INSULIN   +
ADP   +
FAD
NAD

GLYCOGEN SYNTHASE
BUILDS 1,4

BRANCHING:
CUT 1,4
ADD 1,6

GLYCOGEN PHOSPHORYLASE:
CUTS 1,4

DEBRANCHING:
CUT 1,4
ADD 1,4

CUT 1,6 ─OH

5 6
4   1
3 2

NOTES

Metabolism

Glycogen Storage Diseases

TYPE—EPONYM	ORGAN	ENZYME	ACCUMULATION	GLYCOGEN	SXS
I VON GIERKE	HEPATIC	GLUC-6 PHOSPHA	(+)	NORMAL	HUGE LIVER MR, DOLL'S EYES SHORT LIMBS
II POMPE	H/M	LYSOSOMAL 1,4 GLUCOSIDASE	VACUOLES INCLUSION BODIES	NORMAL	HYPO BG HYPOTONIA DEATH BY 2
(L) III CORI (MILD)	H/M	DEBRANCHING	MILD	MANY BRANCHES, SHORT	MILD HYPO BG MILD HYPOTONIA
IV ANDERSON	H/M	BRANCHING	∅	LONG CHAINS 5 BRANCHES	HYPOTONIA CIRRHOSIS DEATH
(L) V MCARDLES	MUSCLE	GLYCOGEN PHOSPHORYLASE	(+)	NORMAL	CRAMPS WEAKNESS MYOGLOBIN
VI HERS	HEPATIC	GLYCOGEN PHOSPHORYLASE	(+)	NORMAL	HYPOGLYCEMIA CIRRHOSIS DEATH BY 2

Lipid Synthesis

Metabolism

Triglyceride Mobilization

ADIPOSE

DHAP ⇐ GLUCOSE

GLYCEROL-3-P *
DEHYDROGENASE

GLYCEROL-3-P + FA

C C C -P

TRIGLYCERIDES

C C C — GLYCEROL BACKBONE

C C C P — INOSITOL — LIPOPHILIC

LIVER

GLUCOSE

GLUCOSE → DHAP

GLYCEROL KINASE

IDL

GLYCEROL → GLYCEROL-3-P
+
FA

LIPOPROTEIN LIPASE

VLDL

FA SYNTHESIS

ACETYL-COA

20%

80%

A₁ SRB2

LCAT HDL ⇄ CETP
HDL

LDL

VLDL REMNANT (IDL)

VLDL B100

HDL

HDL

CHYLOMICRONS B48

E → B48 / CII

E VLDL B100 CII   E CHYLOMICRON REMNANT CII   E CHYLOMICRON B48 C II

LIPOPROTEIN LIPASE

LDL   IDL   VLDL

Lipid Catabolism

ADIPOSE

GLUCOSE

GLYCEROL-3-P

GLYCEROL
+
FA

ALBUMIN

HORMONE SENSITIVE LIPASE

TRIGLYCERIDES

INSULIN

FA
ADIPOSE   MUSCLE
KETONES   GLYCEROL
ATP
ACETYL COA
FA   GLUCOSE

LIVER

GLUCOSE → DHAP
GLYCEROL → GLYC-3-P

FA
ACETYL-COA

MCAD DEF
- HYPO BG
- Ø KETONES FAST
↓ ACYL-TRANS

FA + COA → FATTY ACYL-COA
ATP   ADP
COA
INACTIVE   ACTIVE

CARBOXYLASE
3c   4c
PROPIONYL COA   METHYL MALONYL COA
MUTASE
↑MYELIN
4c SUCCINYL COA
GLUCONEO
B12 DEF

CYTOPLASM

FA

OUTER

CARNITINE ACYL-TRANSFERASE I
FATTY ACYL COA SYTHETASE

INTER MEMBRANE
FA CARNITINE
FA-COA   AMP+P ATP   FA
COA   COA

INNER
CARNITINE
COA
CARNITINE ACYL-TRANS II
FATTY ACYL DEHYDROGENASE

MITOCHONDRIA

FA CARNITINE
COA
FA   EVERY 2-C   2c ACETYL-COA
NAD FAD FADH NADH 3 ATP

LCAD: ≥ 10
MCAD: 6-8
2 ATP

9
2
5
17 ATP
×7
119 ATP

3 NADH
1 FADH₂   TCA
1 GTP

ETC

ATP

Metabolism

HEPATOCYTE

FA OXIDIZE
ACETYL COA
HMG COA SYNTHASE
HMG-COA
HMG COA LYASE
ACETONE
ACETOACETATE (4c)
NADH
NAD
* β-OH-BUTYRATE

THIOPHORASE → ACETOACETYL-COA → 2x ACETYL COA
ACETOACETATE(4)
NAD
NADH
β-OH-BUTYRATE

TCA
ETC
HEP GLYCOGEN   PROTEIN CATABOLISM   FAT CATABOLISM
GLUC
KET

1 2 3 4   1 2 3 4
DAYS   WEEKS

KETOSIS = KETOACIDOSIS
KETONES: URINE/BLOOD SMELL SWEET
ACIDOSIS: AG MET ACID
PH <7.4, BICARB ↓

DKA ↑BG, ⊕ KETONES
PH<7.2

KETONES   ATP   GLYCEROL
ACETYL-COA
FA   GLUCOSE

KETONE DONOR: LIVER
GLYCOGEN
GLUCOSE-6-P
PEP
PYRUVATE
PYRUVATE
ACETYL-COA
ATP TCA ETC NADH ACETYL-COA KETONES

RBC ADIPOSE MUSCLE BRAIN
KETONE RECIPIENT: LIVER
GLUCOSE
GLYCOGEN
GLUCOSE-6-P
PYRUVATE
PYRUVATE
ACETYL-COA
TCA-ETC
KETONES
TCA-ETC

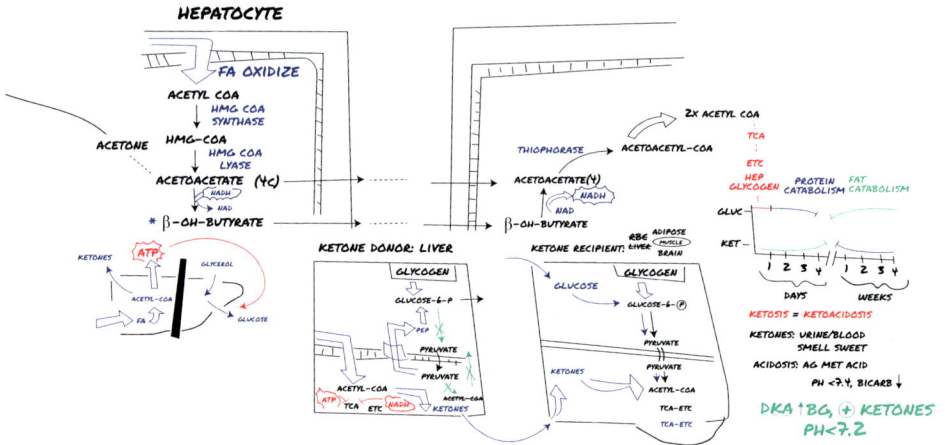

Sphingolipids

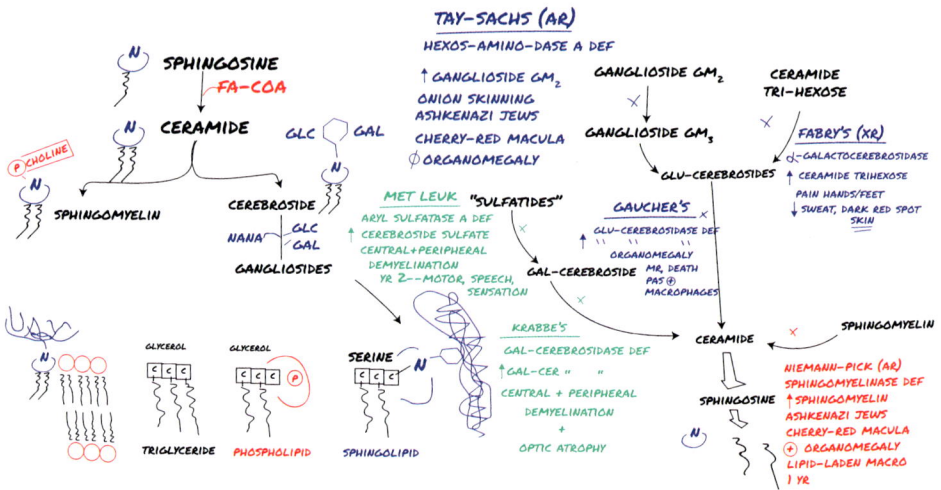

SPHINGOSINE
FA-COA
CERAMIDE
GLC   GAL
P CHOLINE
SPHINGOMYELIN
CEREBROSIDE
NANA   GLC GAL
GANGLIOSIDES

TAY-SACHS (AR)
HEXOS-AMINO-DASE A DEF
↑ GANGLIOSIDE GM₂
ONION SKINNING
ASHKENAZI JEWS
CHERRY-RED MACULA
∅ ORGANOMEGALY

GANGLIOSIDE GM₂
✕
GANGLIOSIDE GM₃
✕
GLU-CEREBROSIDES

CERAMIDE TRI-HEXOSE
✕
FABRY'S (XR)
α-GALACTOCEREBROSIDASE
↑ CERAMIDE TRIHEXOSE
PAIN HANDS/FEET
↓ SWEAT, DARK RED SPOT SKIN

MET LEUK   "SULFATIDES"
ARYL SULFATASE A DEF
↑ CEREBROSIDE SULFATE
CENTRAL+PERIPHERAL DEMYELINATION
YR 2 -- MOTOR, SPEECH, SENSATION

GAUCHER'S
GLU-CEREBROSIDASE DEF
✕
ORGANOMEGALY
MR, DEATH
PAS ⊕
MACROPHAGES
GAL-CEREBROSIDE

CERAMIDE
✕   SPHINGOMYELIN

KRABBE'S
GAL-CEREBROSIDASE DEF
↑ GAL-CER "   "
CENTRAL + PERIPHERAL DEMYELINATION
+
OPTIC ATROPHY

SPHINGOSINE

NIEMANN-PICK (AR)
SPHINGOMYELINASE DEF
↑ SPHINGOMYELIN
ASHKENAZI JEWS
CHERRY-RED MACULA
⊕ ORGANOMEGALY
LIPID-LADEN MACRO
1 YR

GLYCEROL   GLYCEROL   SERINE
C C C   C C C P   C C C   N
TRIGLYCERIDE   PHOSPHOLIPID   SPHINGOLIPID

Metabolism

Excess Nitrogen Metabolism

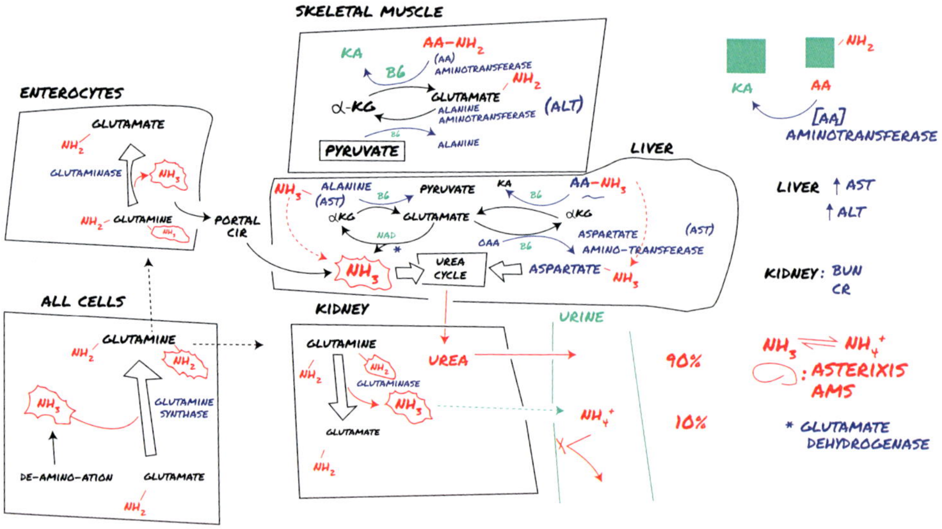

SKELETAL MUSCLE

KA   AA—NH₂
(AA)
B6   AMINOTRANSFERASE
α-KG   NH₂
GLUTAMATE   (ALT)
ALANINE
AMINOTRANSFERASE
PYRUVATE   B6   ALANINE

ENTEROCYTES

GLUTAMATE
NH₂
GLUTAMINASE   NH₃

NH₂ — GLUTAMINE   NH₃   PORTAL CIR

LIVER

NH₃   ALANINE (AST)   PYRUVATE   KA   AA—NH₃
B6   αKG   GLUTAMATE   B6   αKG
NAD   *   OAA   B6   ASPARTATE   (AST)
AMINO-TRANSFERASE
NH₃   UREA CYCLE   ASPARTATE   NH₃

ALL CELLS

GLUTAMINE
NH₂
NH₃
GLUTAMINE SYNTHASE
DE—AMINO—ATION   GLUTAMATE
NH₂

KIDNEY

GLUTAMINE   UREA
NH₂
GLUTAMINASE
NH₃
GLUTAMATE
NH₂

URINE

UREA → 90%

NH₄⁺ → 10%

KA   NH₂
AA
[AA]
AMINOTRANSFERASE

LIVER ↑ AST
↑ ALT

KIDNEY: BUN
CR

$NH_3 \rightleftharpoons NH_4^+$
: ASTERIXIS
AMS

* GLUTAMATE
DEHYDROGENASE

Urea Cycle

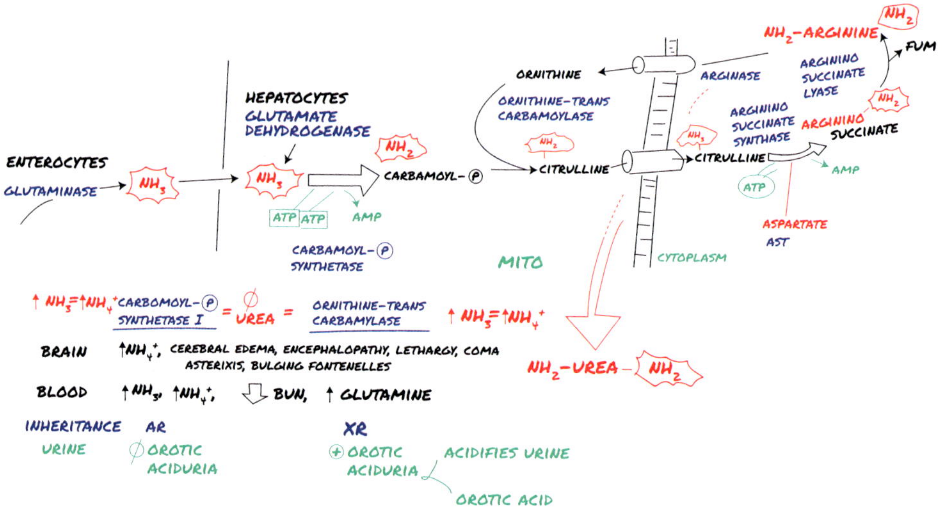

HEPATOCYTES
GLUTAMATE
DEHYDROGENASE

ENTEROCYTES

GLUTAMINASE → NH₃   NH₃   NH₂
CARBAMOYL—Ⓟ → CITRULLINE
ATP ATP   AMP

CARBAMOYL—Ⓟ
SYNTHETASE

ORNITHINE
ORNITHINE—TRANS
CARBAMYLASE
NH₂

CITRULLINE

NH₂—ARGININE   NH₂
FUM
ARGININO
SUCCINATE
LYASE
ARGININO   ARGININO   NH₂
SUCCINATE   SUCCINATE
SYNTHASE
ATP   AMP
ASPARTATE
AST

MITO   CYTOPLASM

NH₂—UREA — NH₂

$\uparrow NH_3 \rightleftharpoons \uparrow NH_4^+$ CARBAMOYL—Ⓟ   ∅
SYNTHETASE I   = UREA =   ORNITHINE—TRANS $\uparrow NH_3 \rightleftharpoons \uparrow NH_4^+$
CARBAMYLASE

BRAIN   ↑NH₄⁺, CEREBRAL EDEMA, ENCEPHALOPATHY, LETHARGY, COMA
ASTERIXIS, BULGING FONTENELLES

BLOOD   ↑NH₃, ↑NH₄⁺,   ⇩ BUN,   ↑ GLUTAMINE

INHERITANCE   AR   XR
URINE   ∅ OROTIC   ⊕ OROTIC   ACIDIFIES URINE
ACIDURIA   ACIDURIA

OROTIC ACID

Metabolism

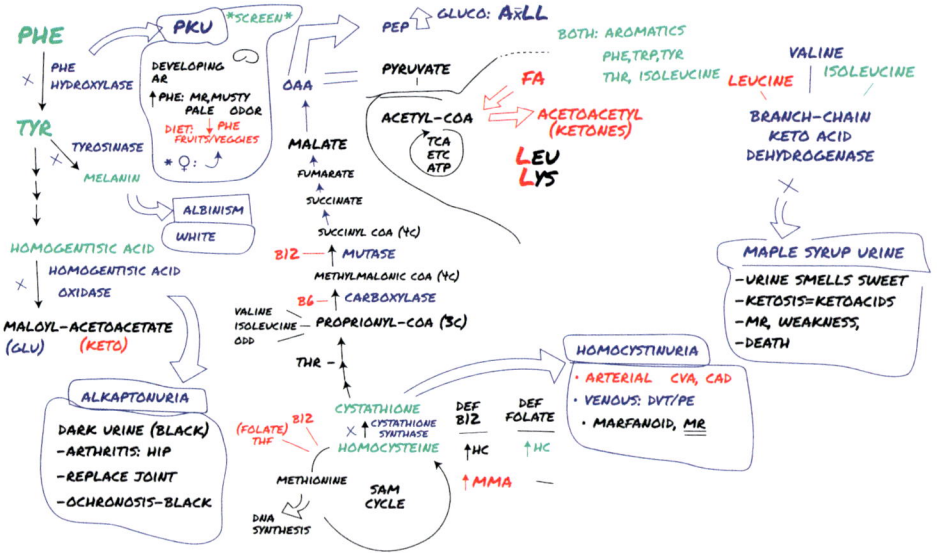

Metabolism

Intro to Genetics

CENTROMERE

CHR 1
2 CHROMOSOMES
2 COPIES

CHR 1
2 CHROMOSOMES
4 COPIES
2 CHROMATID PER CHR

LOCUS

(GENE 1)
GENE
ALLELE

(GENE 1) V1
ALLELE

(GENE 1) V2
ALLELE

GENE V1 + GENE V2

ALLELE 1   ALLELE 2

CODE   GENOTYPE

HOMO
A1, A1

HETERO
A1, A2

HOMO
A2, A2

S/S   PHENOTYPE

DOMINANT = GAIN FXN
1 COPY=ACTIVE
5X5 ⊕ 1 COPY ⊕

RECESSIVE = LOSS OF FXN
LOSS OF BOTH COPIES

META CENTRIC

SUB META CENTRIC

ACRO CENTRIC

P

*ROBERTSONIAN

CHR 1

CHR 22

X,Y
23

AUTOSOMAL

2N

4N

2N

N

G_1
SYNTHESIS

MEIOSIS I

MEIOSIS II

MEIOSIS II

1   8   1   8

TRANSLOCATION
RECOMBINATION
EXCHANGE

CHR 1 G_2

M

G_1

CHR 1

S

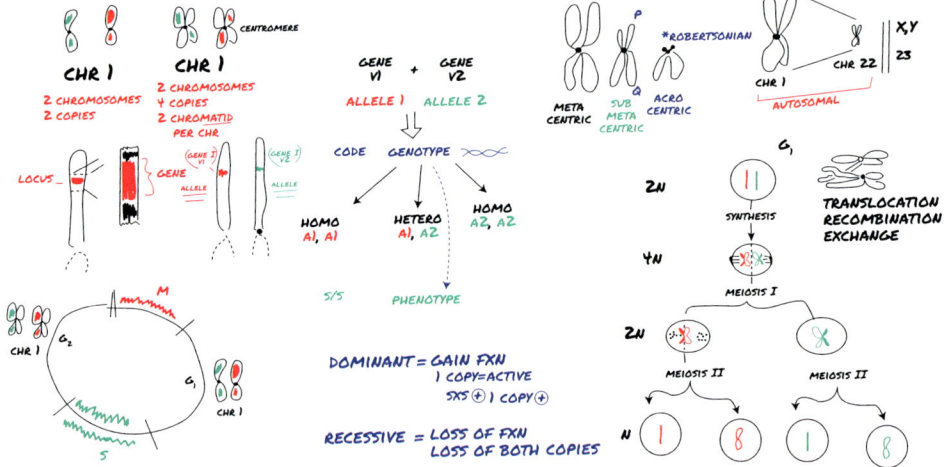

Modes of Inheritance

	♂ → ♂ (FATHER) (SON)	GENERATION		CARRIER	RECURRENCE
AD (GENDER NEUTRAL)	⊕	EVERY		—	50% ONE AFFECTED ~~75% BOTH AFFECTED~~
AR	⊕	SKIPS		BOTH PARENTS OBLIGATE CARRIERS NEXT CHILD: 50% ~~CHILD'S DZ: 66%~~	25% (BOTH CARRIERS)
XD (MEN ONLY)	⊖	EVERY		—	♂ (⊗) : 100% DAUGHT 50% KIDS 0% SONS ♀ (⊗) : 50% KIDS ♂ = ♀
XR	⊖	SKIPS		OBLIGATE DAUGHTERS MOTHERS AFFECTED MALES	25% OF ALL BIRTHS 100% AFFECTED= ♂
MITOCHONDRIAL	ALL OF MOM'S KIDS				

Genetics

Complexities of Inheritance

INCOMPLETE PENETRANCE

GENOTYPE ⊕   SHOULD HAVE DZ

PHENOTYPE ∅ △   BUT THEY DON'T

BRCA-1/2   80% PENETRANCE

VARIABLE EXPRESSION

GENOTYPE ⊕   SHOULD HAVE DZ

PHENOTYPE ⊕   AND YOU DO

EVERY DISEASE

NATURE   NURTURE

ANTICIPATION

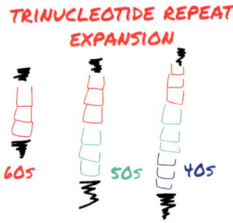

TRINUCLEOTIDE REPEAT EXPANSION

60s   50s   40s

IMPRINTING

METHYLATION = INACTIVATES

♂   ♀

$\frac{x}{2}$ → PW
$\frac{x}{3}$

ANGELMAN ← $\frac{x}{3}$

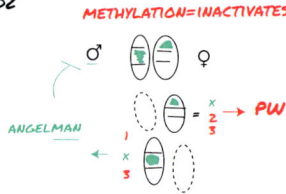

NEW MUTATIONS

POST-FERTILIZATION MOSAICSM

BABY'S FAULT
↳ 0% RECURRENCE

PLEIOTROPY

GENOTYPE ⊕ → PHENO → PHENO → PHENO

MARFAN

LOCUS HETERO

CHR 7 → OI ← CHR 17

Population Genetics Math

	P	Q
P	P^2 NORMAL	PQ CARRIER
Q	PQ CARRIER	Q^2 AFFECTED

(OI + OII + OIII = 1)

$$P^2 + 2PQ + Q^2 = 1$$

GENOTYPE FREQ

$$P + Q = 1$$

ALLELE FREQ

GENOTYPE ⟷ ALLELE

16 IN 100 ARE AFFECTED
PREVALENCE

$\frac{16}{100} = Q^2$

$\frac{.4}{(40\%)} = \frac{4}{10} = Q$

$\frac{.6}{(60\%)} = \frac{6}{10} = P$

$P^2 \; 2PQ \; Q^2 \; // \; P \; Q$ FREQUENCIES (%)

GENOTYPE X #
ALLELE X # X 2

OI : $P^2 = .36$ NORMAL

OII : $2PQ = .48$ CARRIER

OIII : $Q^2 = .16$ AFFECTED

1.00

X-LINKED RECESSIVE

Q = RATE OF AFFECTED

Q = OIII

CTRL	OI	OII	OIII

SOUTHERN

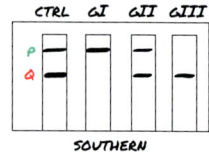

GENOTYPE ⟷ ALLELE   RARE (AR)

CARRIER
AFFECTED

1 IN 10,000 ARE AFFECTED

$\frac{1}{10,000} = Q^2$

$\frac{.01}{(1\%)} = \frac{1}{100} = Q$

$1 \approx P$

1 IN 50 ARE CARRIERS

$\frac{1}{50} = 2PQ = 2Q$

$\frac{1}{100} = Q$

$Q^2 = 1$

$(2)(1)(Q) = \frac{2}{100} = \frac{1}{50}$

$P^2 = \frac{1}{10,000}$

.

Population Genetics Concepts

NEW MUTATION

- EVOLVE... SPECIES
  - ↳ NEVER SEE
- SPONTANEOUSLY RARELY, SLOW, UNDETECTABLE
- INDUCED FAST, ABUNDANT, HARMFUL (RADIATION)

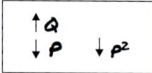

$$\uparrow Q \quad \downarrow P \quad \downarrow P^2$$

RECOMBINATION

- NO △ DNA
- REDISTRIBUTION OF TRAITS (GAMETES)
- ALWAYS BAD (SOMATIC)   ∅△Q

ONCOGENE=GAIN FXN=CANCER (BCR-ABL)

TUMOR SUPPRESSOR= LOSS FXN=CANCER (P53)

NATURAL SELECTION

GENETICS ADAPTED FOR SURVIVAL PERSIST

AR... ↓Q ...... ↑Q c̄ MEDS

SICKLE CELL →
- P^2-PP-HGBA$_2$ → DIES FROM MALARIA
- PQ HGBSC = 1/10 AA vs. 1/3 A AFRICA
- Q^2-QQ-HGB SS = DIES FROM SICKLE CELL

∅Q̶

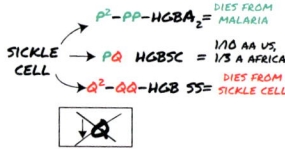

GENETIC DRIFT

SMALL POPULATION
∅ STATS (N)

NEW MUTATION

FOUNDER EFFECT

↓↑Q

GENE FLOW

LARGE POPULATIONS MIX

AA: HGBSS   CF

CA: HGBSS   CF

MIX HGBSS   CF

↓Q   ↓↓Q²

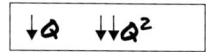

CONSANGUINITY   ↑Q ↑↑Q²

SMALL POPULATION
MATE INTERNALLY
COEFFICIENT OF CONSANGUINITY
PARENT + CHILD 1/2
CHILD + CHILD 1/2
SIBLING-PARENT + CHILD 1/4
1ST COUSINS 1/8
2ND COUSINS 1/32

Chromosome Number Diseases

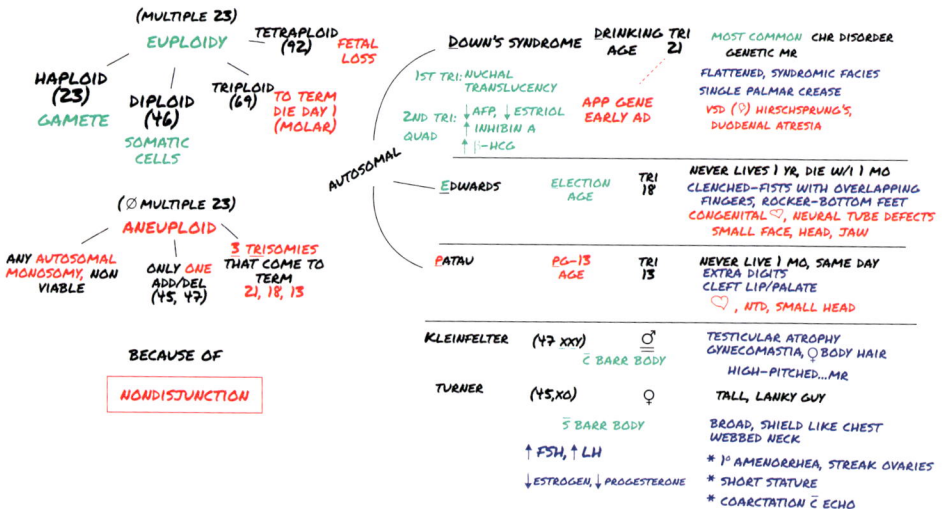

(MULTIPLE 23)
EUPLOIDY — TETRAPLOID (92) FETAL LOSS

HAPLOID (23) GAMETE

DIPLOID (46) SOMATIC CELLS

TRIPLOID (69) TO TERM DIE DAY 1 (MOLAR)

AUTOSOMAL

DOWN'S SYNDROME — DRINKING TRI AGE 21

1ST TRI: NUCHAL TRANSLUCENCY

2ND TRI: ↓AFP, ↓ESTRIOL
↑ INHIBIN A
↑ β-HCG
QUAD

APP GENE EARLY AD

MOST COMMON CHR DISORDER GENETIC MR
FLATTENED, SYNDROMIC FACIES
SINGLE PALMAR CREASE
VSD (♡) HIRSCHSPRUNG'S, DUODENAL ATRESIA

EDWARDS — ELECTION AGE — TRI 18

NEVER LIVES 1 YR, DIE W/1 MO
CLENCHED-FISTS WITH OVERLAPPING FINGERS, ROCKER-BOTTOM FEET
CONGENITAL ♡, NEURAL TUBE DEFECTS
SMALL FACE, HEAD, JAW

PATAU — PG-13 AGE — TRI 13

NEVER LIVE 1 MO, SAME DAY
EXTRA DIGITS
CLEFT LIP/PALATE
♡, NTD, SMALL HEAD

(∅ MULTIPLE 23)
ANEUPLOID

ANY AUTOSOMAL MONOSOMY, NON VIABLE

ONLY ONE ADD/DEL (45, 47)

3 TRISOMIES THAT COME TO TERM 21, 18, 13

BECAUSE OF

NONDISJUNCTION

KLEINFELTER (47 XXY) ♂ c̄ BARR BODY

TESTICULAR ATROPHY
GYNECOMASTIA, ♀ BODY HAIR
HIGH-PITCHED...MR

TURNER (45,XO) ♀ s̄ BARR BODY

TALL, LANKY GUY

BROAD, SHIELD LIKE CHEST WEBBED NECK

↑ FSH, ↑ LH

↓ESTROGEN, ↓ PROGESTERONE

* 1° AMENORRHEA, STREAK OVARIES
* SHORT STATURE
* COARCTATION c̄ ECHO

NOTES

Genetics

Chromosome Structure Diseases

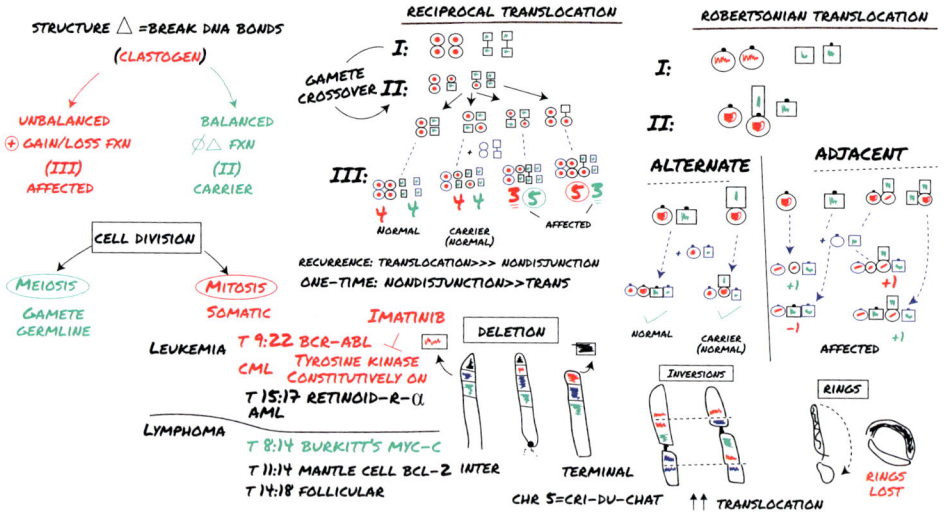

STRUCTURE △ =BREAK DNA BONDS
(CLASTOGEN)

UNBALANCED — BALANCED
⊕ GAIN/LOSS FXN — ∅△ FXN
(III) — (II)
AFFECTED — CARRIER

CELL DIVISION

MEIOSIS — MITOSIS
GAMETE — SOMATIC
GERMLINE

LEUKEMIA — T 9:22 BCR-ABL — IMATINIB
CML — TYROSINE KINASE CONSTITUTIVELY ON
T 15:17 RETINOID-R-α
AML

LYMPHOMA
T 8:14 BURKITT'S MYC-C
T 11:14 MANTLE CELL BCL-2
T 14:18 FOLLICULAR

RECIPROCAL TRANSLOCATION

I:
GAMETE CROSSOVER II:
III:
NORMAL — CARRIER (NORMAL) — AFFECTED

RECURRENCE: TRANSLOCATION>>> NONDISJUNCTION
ONE-TIME: NONDISJUNCTION>>TRANS

DELETION

INTER

TERMINAL

CHR 5=CRI-DU-CHAT ↑↑ TRANSLOCATION

INVERSIONS

ROBERTSONIAN TRANSLOCATION

I:
II:

ALTERNATE — ADJACENT

NORMAL — CARRIER (NORMAL) — AFFECTED

+) +)
-) +)

RINGS
RINGS LOST

Genetics

Plasma Membranes

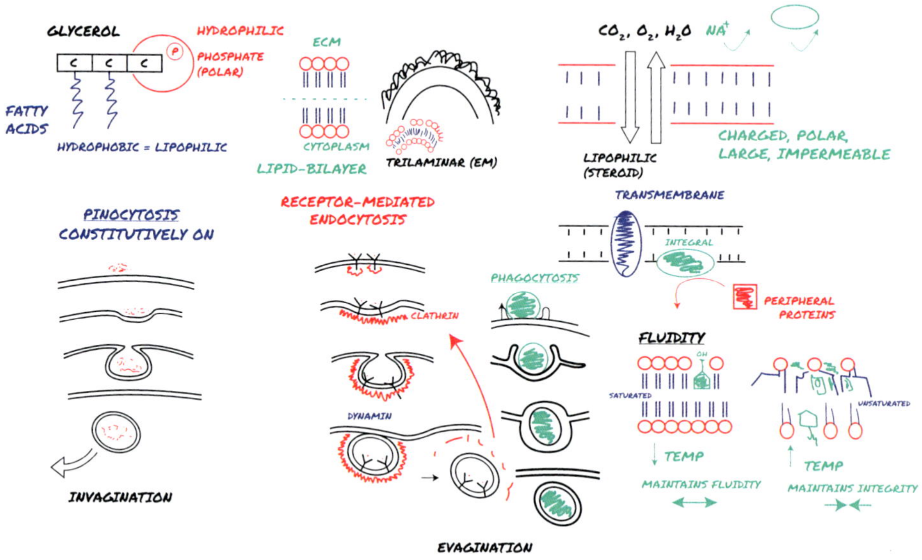

OnlineMedEd

GLYCEROL · HYDROPHILIC · PHOSPHATE (POLAR) · FATTY ACIDS · HYDROPHOBIC = LIPOPHILIC

ECM · CYTOPLASM · LIPID-BILAYER · TRILAMINAR (EM)

CO_2, O_2, H_2O · Na^+ · LIPOPHILIC (STEROID) · CHARGED, POLAR, LARGE, IMPERMEABLE

PINOCYTOSIS CONSTITUTIVELY ON · INVAGINATION

RECEPTOR-MEDIATED ENDOCYTOSIS · CLATHRIN · DYNAMIN · EVAGINATION

TRANSMEMBRANE · INTEGRAL · PHAGOCYTOSIS · PERIPHERAL PROTEINS

FLUIDITY · SATURATED · UNSATURATED · ↓ TEMP · MAINTAINS FLUIDITY · ↑ TEMP · MAINTAINS INTEGRITY

Transporters

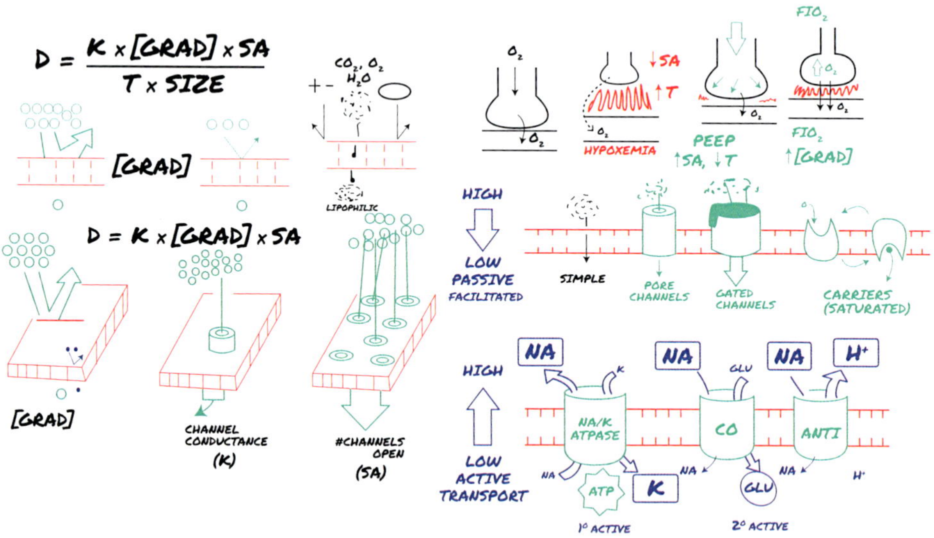

$$D = \frac{K \times [GRAD] \times SA}{T \times SIZE}$$

[GRAD]

$$D = K \times [GRAD] \times SA$$

[GRAD] · CHANNEL CONDUCTANCE (K) · #CHANNELS OPEN (SA)

CO_2, O_2, H_2O · LIPOPHILIC

O_2 · ↓SA ↑T · HYPOXEMIA · PEEP ↑SA, ↓T · FIO_2 ↑[GRAD]

HIGH → LOW PASSIVE FACILITATED · SIMPLE · PORE CHANNELS · GATED CHANNELS · CARRIERS (SATURATED)

HIGH → LOW ACTIVE TRANSPORT

NA · K · NA/K ATPASE · ATP · $1°$ ACTIVE · NA · GLU · CO · K · GLU · NA · H^+ · ANTI · $2°$ ACTIVE

54

© 2020 OnlineMedEd

General Physiology

Membrane-Bound Organelles

SER
SARCOPLASMIC RETICULUM

DETOXIFICATION
LIPID SYNTHESIS

⇩

HEPATOCYTES

RER

SECRETORY
EXOCYTOSIS

LYSOSOME

GOLGI:

CIS: CLOSE TO NUCLEUS
TRANS: PLASMA MEMBRANE
POST-TRANSLATIONAL
   MODIFICATION
SORT + TAG DESTINATION

TRANS
TGN
CIS
G-M-P
COPI
COPII
EARLY ENDOSOME = DECIDE
LATE ENDOSOME
LYSOSOME

VESICLES

⤻ = LYSOZYMES
● = VESICLE
⤳ = ENDOSOME

CYTO
ENDO
ENDO
LAMINA
NUCLEUS

MITO
TCA/ETC = OXIDATIVE
               PHOSPHORYLATION

CYTC = APOPTOSIS

DOUBLE LIPID BILAYER

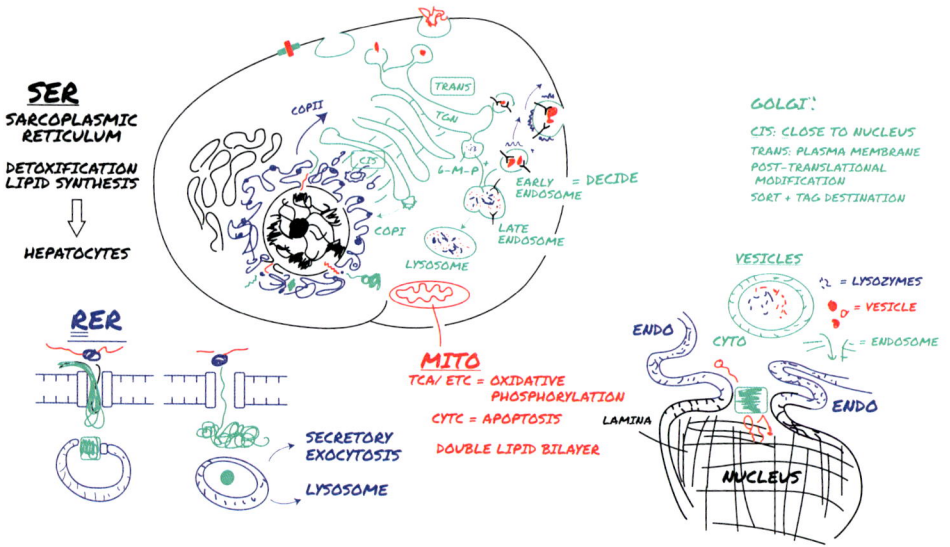

Cytoskeleton

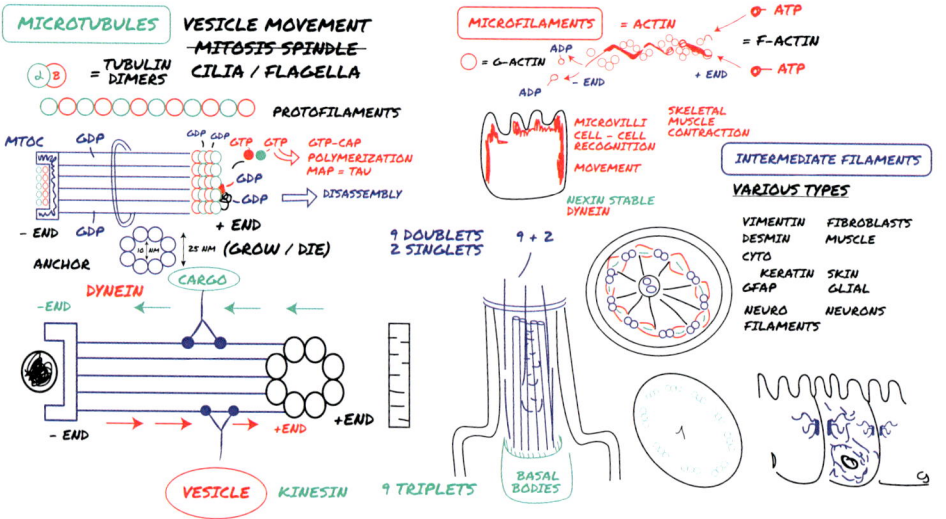

MICROTUBULES

VESICLE MOVEMENT
~~MITOSIS SPINDLE~~
CILIA / FLAGELLA

α β = TUBULIN DIMERS

PROTOFILAMENTS

MTOC   GDP
GDP GDP GTP GTP GTP-CAP
                  POLYMERIZATION
          GDP   MAP = TAU
          GDP
          GDP   ⇨ DISASSEMBLY
- END GDP   + END
ANCHOR   25 NM (GROW / DIE)
           10 NM

DYNEIN
CARGO
-END ←
- END → +END +END
VESICLE   KINESIN

9 DOUBLETS
2 SINGLETS

9 + 2

9 TRIPLETS

BASAL BODIES

MICROFILAMENTS = ACTIN   ● ATP

● = G-ACTIN   = F-ACTIN
ADP   ● ATP
     ADP   ● = END + END

MICROVILLI   SKELETAL
CELL - CELL   MUSCLE
RECOGNITION   CONTRACTION

MOVEMENT

NEXIN STABLE
DYNEIN

INTERMEDIATE FILAMENTS

VARIOUS TYPES

VIMENTIN   FIBROBLASTS
DESMIN   MUSCLE
CYTO
   KERATIN   SKIN
GFAP   GLIAL
NEURO   NEURONS
FILAMENTS

General Physiology

Receptors

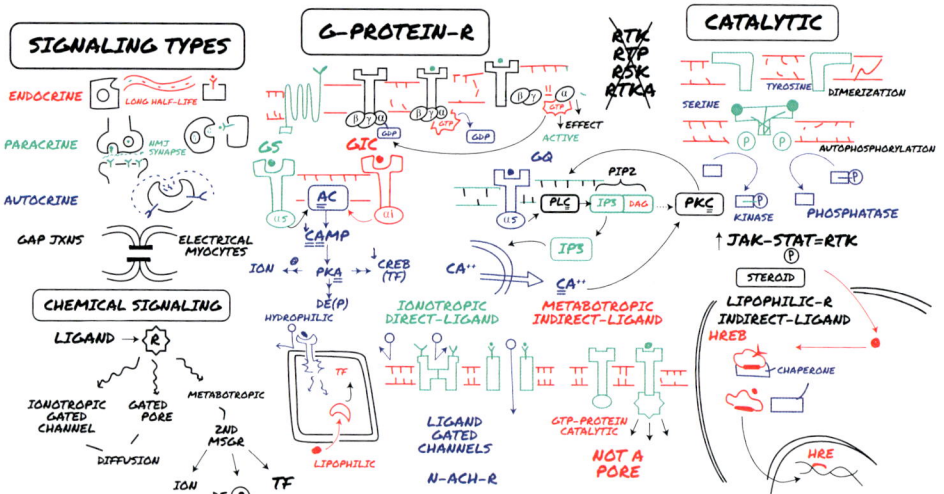

SIGNALING TYPES

ENDOCRINE — LONG HALF-LIFE

PARACRINE — NMJ SYNAPSE

AUTOCRINE

GAP JXNS — ELECTRICAL MYOCYTES

CHEMICAL SIGNALING

LIGAND → R

IONOTROPIC GATED CHANNEL — GATED PORE — METABOTROPIC — 2ND MSGR

DIFFUSION — ION — DE(P) — TF

LIPOPHILIC

G-PROTEIN-R

GS — GIC — GQ

AC — cAMP

ION — PKA — CREB (TF)

DE(P) — HYDROPHILIC

PIP2 — PLC — IP3 — DAG — PKC

IP3 — CA⁺⁺

CA⁺⁺

IONOTROPIC DIRECT-LIGAND

LIGAND GATED CHANNELS — N-ACH-R

METABOTROPIC INDIRECT-LIGAND

GTP-PROTEIN CATALYTIC

NOT A PORE

GDP — GTP — EFFECT — ACTIVE

RTK RTP RSK RTKA

CATALYTIC

SERINE — TYROSINE — DIMERIZATION

P — P — AUTOPHOSPHORYLATION

KINASE — PHOSPHATASE

↑ JAK-STAT=RTK (P)

STEROID

LIPOPHILIC-R INDIRECT-LIGAND

HREB — CHAPERONE

HRE

Excitable Cells: Passive Properties

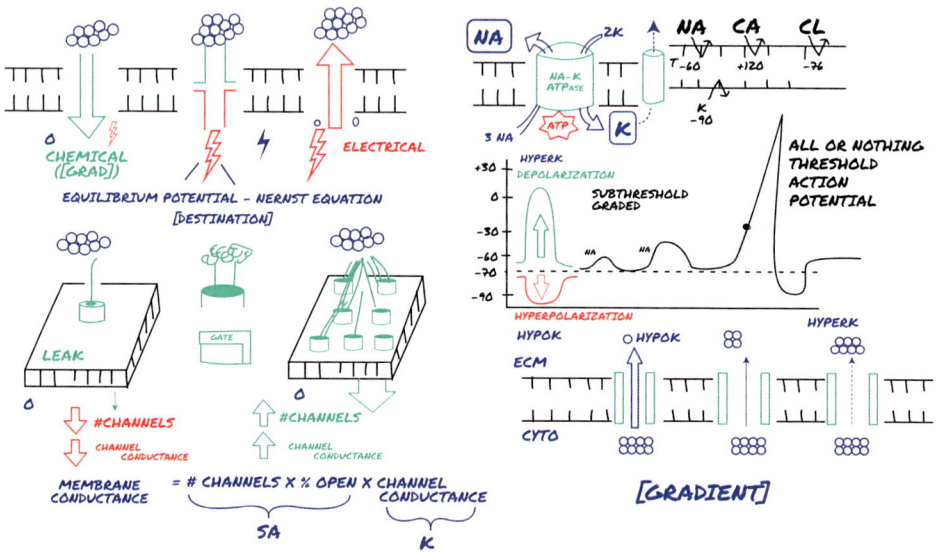

CHEMICAL ([GRAD]) — ELECTRICAL

EQUILIBRIUM POTENTIAL - NERNST EQUATION [DESTINATION]

LEAK

↓ #CHANNELS — ↓ CHANNEL CONDUCTANCE

↑ #CHANNELS — ↑ CHANNEL CONDUCTANCE

MEMBRANE CONDUCTANCE = # CHANNELS X % OPEN X CHANNEL CONDUCTANCE

SA — K

NA — 2K — NA-K ATPase — K

3 NA — ATP

	NA	CA	CL
	-60	+120	-76

K -90

HYPERK — DEPOLARIZATION

SUBTHRESHOLD GRADED

+30, 0, -30, -60, -70, -90

NA — NA

HYPERPOLARIZATION

ALL OR NOTHING THRESHOLD ACTION POTENTIAL

HYPOK — HYPOK — HYPERK

ECM

CYTO

[GRADIENT]

General Physiology

Excitable Cells: Active Properties

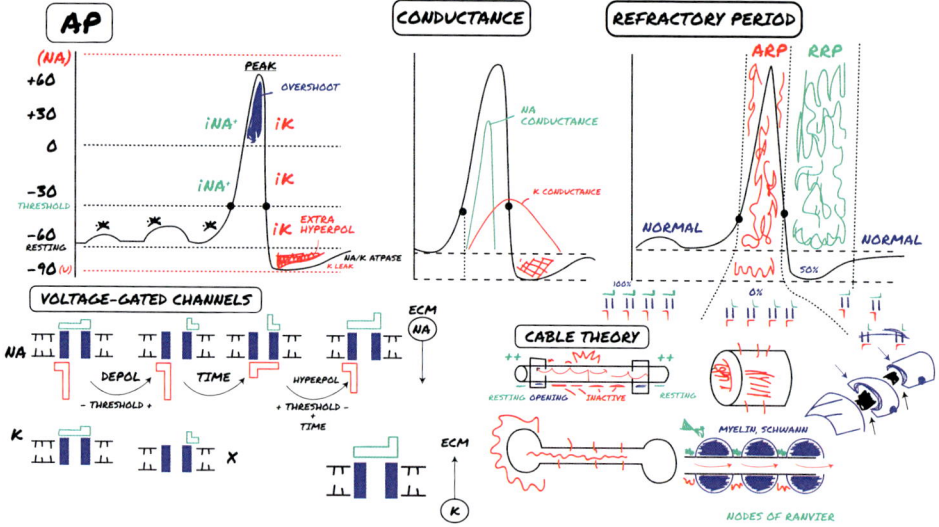

Synapses

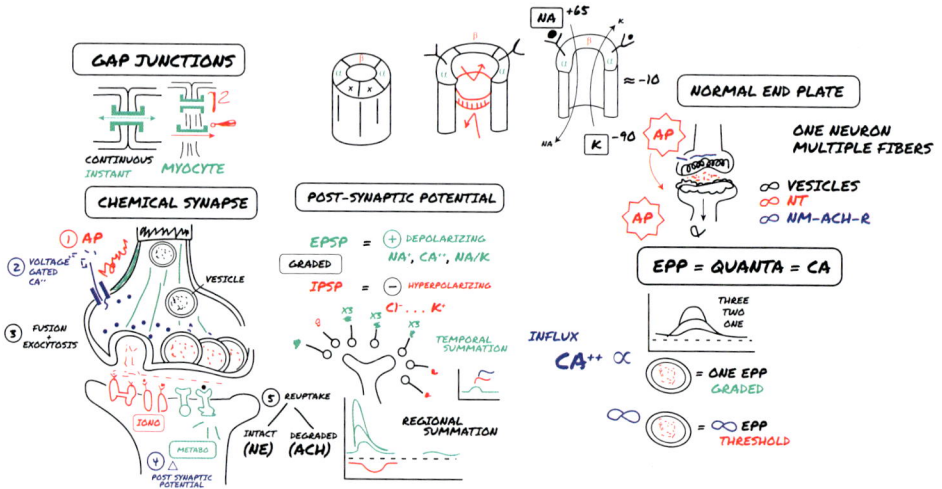

NOTES

Epithelium

POLARITY

APICAL
LAT — □ — LAT
BASAL
BM

DESCRIBE

#LAYERS
- SIMPLE = 1 LAYER
- STRATIFIED >1 LAYER

SIZE + SHAPE
- COLUMNAR H>W
- CUBOID H=W
- SQUAMOUS W>H

SPECIAL
- PSEUDO STRATIFIED
- TRANSITIONAL UROGENITAL

FXN

NONMOTILE CILIA 9+0

APICAL
- MICROVILLI – ACTIN – ⬆SA – ⬆ABSORPTION
  GUT (STRIATED) KIDNEY (BRUSH)
- STEREOCILIA – ACTIN – LONG MICROVILLI
  MECHANORECEPTORS EAR
- CILIA
  FLAGELLA – MT, BASAL BODY, AXONEME   DYNEIN
  9 TRIP   9 DBLS+2 SING, –END

TALKING + ADHESION

LATERAL
- ZONA OCCLUDENS – "PLUGS LEAKS"
  → TIGHT JXNS = ⬇PARACELLULAR
  → LOCKS APEX   CLAUDINS, OCCLUDINS
- MACULA ADHERENS   ZONA ADHERENS – "BUMP + CONTROL"
  → INTRA ACTIN → EXTRA CAM – E-CADHERIN
                                  INTEGRIN
                                  FIBRONECTIN
- DESMOSOMES = SPOT-WELDS   INTRA INTERMEDIATE
                              EXTRA DESMOGLEIN, DESMOCOLLIN

ANCHOR + PROTECT

BASAL
FOCAL ADHESIONS ACTIN   HEMIDESMOSOMES

TYPE VII COL
FIBRILLIN
FIBRILS
ELASTIN
LAMINA DENSA = BASAL LAMINA
RETICULAR LAMINA

DOME-SHAPED
SQUAMOUS

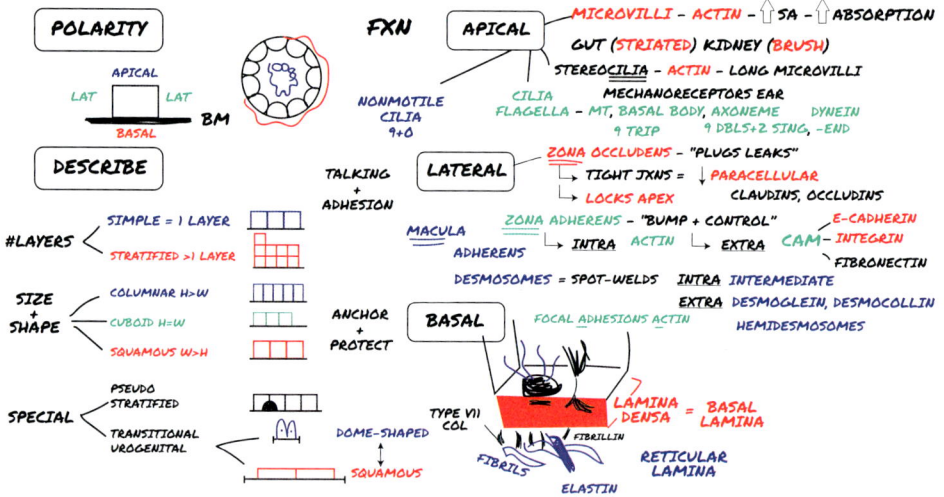

Neuromuscular Diseases

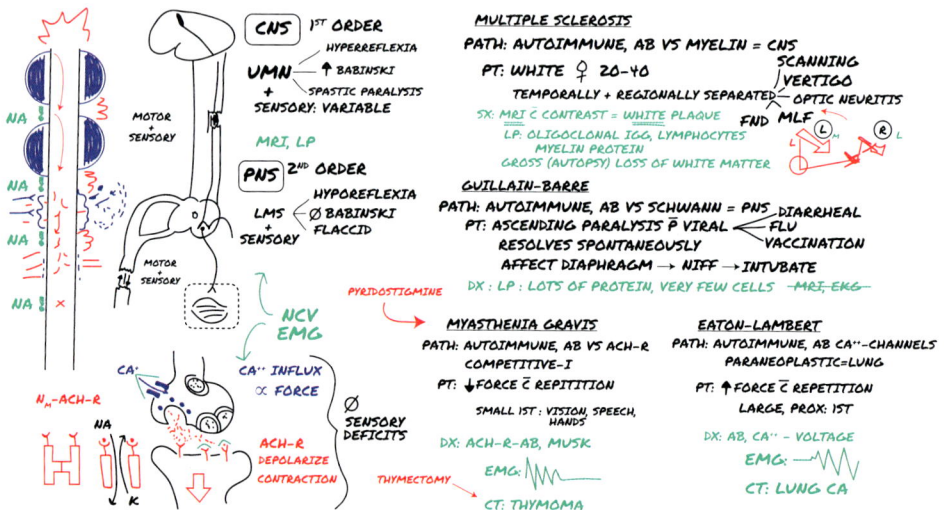

CNS 1ST ORDER
UMN
- HYPERREFLEXIA
- ⬆BABINSKI
- SPASTIC PARALYSIS
+ SENSORY: VARIABLE

MRI, LP

PNS 2ND ORDER
LMN
- HYPOREFLEXIA
- Ø BABINSKI
- FLACCID
+ SENSORY

NA
NA
NA
NA ×

MOTOR + SENSORY

MOTOR SENSORY

NCV EMG

CA⁺⁺ INFLUX ∝ FORCE

Ø SENSORY DEFICITS

N_M-ACH-R
NA
NA
K

ACH-R DEPOLARIZE CONTRACTION

PYRIDOSTIGMINE

THYMECTOMY

MULTIPLE SCLEROSIS
PATH: AUTOIMMUNE, AB VS MYELIN = CNS
PT: WHITE ♀ 20-40
  TEMPORALLY + REGIONALLY SEPARATED
  SCANNING
  VERTIGO
  OPTIC NEURITIS
  FND MLF
SX: MRI c̄ CONTRAST = WHITE PLAQUE
  LP: OLIGOCLONAL IGG, LYMPHOCYTES
      MYELIN PROTEIN
  GROSS (AUTOPSY) LOSS OF WHITE MATTER

L ——— R
L

GUILLAIN-BARRE
PATH: AUTOIMMUNE, AB VS SCHWANN = PNS
PT: ASCENDING PARALYSIS p̄ VIRAL
  DIARRHEAL
  FLU
  VACCINATION
  RESOLVES SPONTANEOUSLY
  AFFECT DIAPHRAGM → NIFF → INTUBATE
DX: LP : LOTS OF PROTEIN, VERY FEW CELLS   MRI, EKG

MYASTHENIA GRAVIS
PATH: AUTOIMMUNE, AB VS ACH-R
  COMPETITIVE-I
PT: ⬇FORCE c̄ REPETITION
  SMALL 1ST : VISION, SPEECH, HANDS
DX: ACH-R-AB, MUSK
EMG: 〰️
CT: THYMOMA

EATON-LAMBERT
PATH: AUTOIMMUNE, AB CA⁺⁺-CHANNELS
  PARANEOPLASTIC=LUNG
PT: ⬆FORCE c̄ REPETITION
  LARGE, PROX: 1ST
DX: AB, CA⁺⁺ – VOLTAGE
EMG: 〰️
CT: LUNG CA

General Physiology

Skeletal Muscle

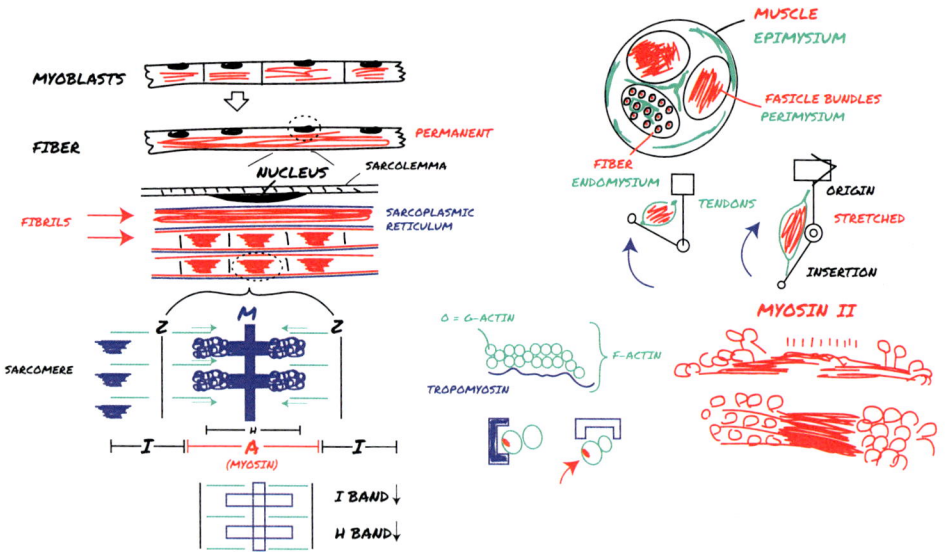

MYOBLASTS

FIBER

PERMANENT

NUCLEUS

SARCOLEMMA

FIBRILS

SARCOPLASMIC RETICULUM

SARCOMERE

Z — M — Z

A (MYOSIN)

I — H — I

I BAND ↓

H BAND ↓

MUSCLE EPIMYSIUM

FASICLE BUNDLES PERIMYSIUM

FIBER ENDOMYSIUM

TENDONS

ORIGIN

STRETCHED

INSERTION

O = G-ACTIN

F-ACTIN

TROPOMYOSIN

MYOSIN II

Excitation, Contraction, Coupling

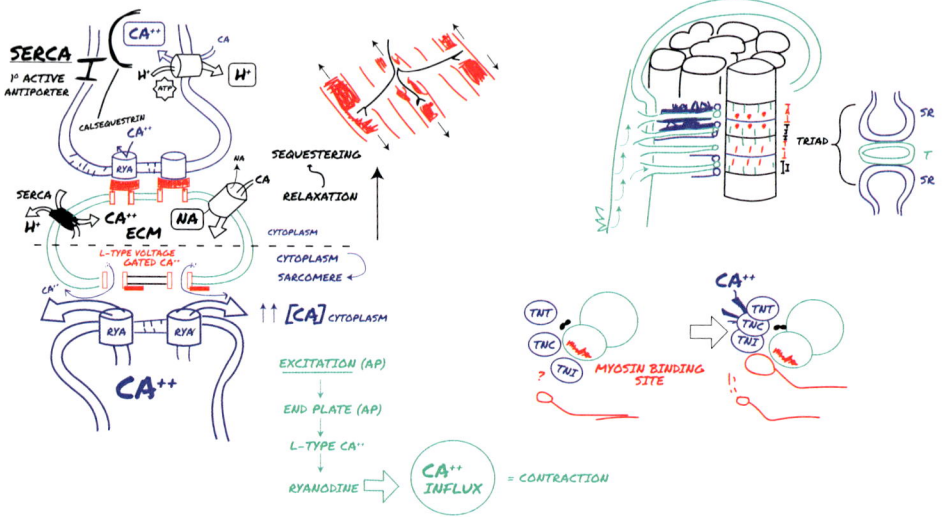

SERCA

1° ACTIVE ANTIPORTER

CA⁺⁺

CA

H^+

H^+

CALSEQUESTRIN

CA⁺⁺

RYA

NA

CA

SEQUESTERING

SERCA

H^+

CA⁺⁺

ECM

NA

RELAXATION

CYTOPLASM

L-TYPE VOLTAGE GATED CA⁺⁺

CYTOPLASM

SARCOMERE

CA⁺⁺

RYA

RYA

↑↑ [CA] CYTOPLASM

CA⁺⁺

EXCITATION (AP)

END PLATE (AP)

L-TYPE CA⁺⁺

RYANODINE

CA⁺⁺ INFLUX

= CONTRACTION

TRIAD

SR

T

SR

CA⁺⁺

TNT

TNC

TNI

? TNI

MYOSIN BINDING SITE

TNT

TNC

TNI

NOTES

Myopathies

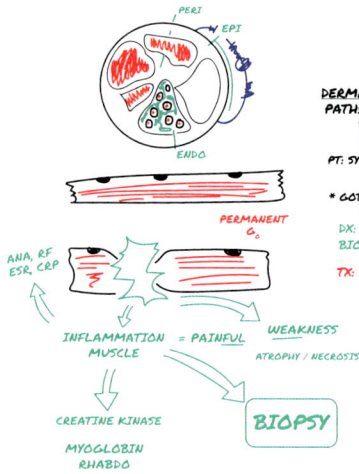

(PAIN) INFLAMMATORY MYOPATHIES (WEAK)

DERMATO – MYO – SITIS
PATH: CD4 → EPIMYSIUM
  CAPILLARIES, SK MUSCLE
  DERMATO (SKIN)
  MYOSITIS (MUSCLE)
PT: SYMMETRIC PROXIMAL
  PAINFUL WEAKNESS
  TENDER MUSCLES
  * GOTTRON'S PAPULES, SHAWL
    SIGN, *HELIOTYPE RASH
DX: ANA → JO, MI2
  BIOPSY → PERIPHERAL
    ATROPHY
TX: STEROIDS

POLYMYOSITIS
CD8 → ENDOMYSIUM

MYOSITIS
SPPW
TM

SA – DM
CENTRAL
NECROSIS
TX: STEROIDS

INCLUSION BODY MYOSITIS
? ?

MYOSITIS
ASYMMETRIC DISTAL
PAINLESS WEAKNESS
>60 "NMJ"

BIOPSY → VACUOLES
  INCLUSION BODIES

TX: N/A

ANA, RF
ESR, CRP

PERMANENT
G₀

INFLAMMATION = PAINFUL
MUSCLE

WEAKNESS
ATROPHY / NECROSIS

CREATINE KINASE
MYOGLOBIN
RHABDO

BIOPSY

DUCHENNE DYSTROPHY
PATH: X–LINKED RECESSIVE
  DYSTROPHIN GENE DELETED
  SK MUSCLE → ADIPOSE

DX: BIOPSY = ADIPOSE . . . GENETIC
TX: SUPPORTIVE

PT: 1 YO
PROXIMAL → DISTAL
PARALYSIS TEENS
DEATH BY 20
CALF PSEUDOHYPERTROPHY
GOWER'S SIGN

BECKER'S
MUTATION
DYSTORPHIN
VARIABLE
♀♂ = NORMAL
  DEATH

Skeletal Muscle Force

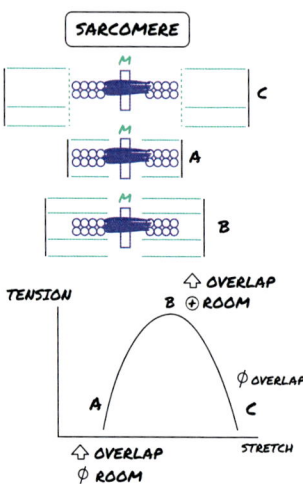

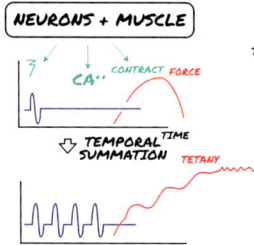

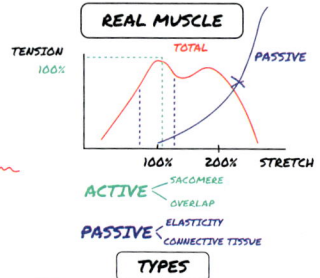

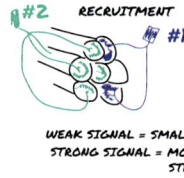

SARCOMERE

C

A

B

TENSION

B ⊕ OVERLAP
  ROOM

φ OVERLAP

A

C

↑ OVERLAP
φ ROOM

STRETCH

NEURONS + MUSCLE

CA⁺⁺

CONTRACT FORCE

TEMPORAL SUMMATION
TIME

TETANY

#2

RECRUITMENT
#1

WEAK SIGNAL = SMALLEST UNIT
STRONG SIGNAL = MORE UNITS
  STEPWISE

REAL MUSCLE

TENSION
100%

TOTAL

PASSIVE

100% 200% STRETCH

ACTIVE < SARCOMERE
  OVERLAP

PASSIVE < ELASTICITY
  CONNECTIVE TISSUE

TYPES

RED
OXIDATIVE ← MITO (ETC)
PHOS   VESSELS
        MYOGLOBIN
GLYCOGEN

SMALL MOTOR UNITS
COORDINATION
SUSTAINED CONTRACTIONS

WHITE
GLYCOLYSIS / ANAEROBIC

GLYCOGEN
LARGE MOTOR
BURST

General Physiology

Smooth Muscle

CA IN

~~SR RUSH, RYAN, AP~~

- HIGHLY DEPENDENT

  [CA] ECM

- CAVEOLAE = "T-TUBULES"

- ⬆ LATENCY ⎫ 10% ATP
- ⬆ DURATION ⎭ OF SK MUSCLE

Gq - PIP2 - IP3 - CA

ARTERIOLAR STRETCH

LIGAND GATED   VOLTAGE GATED

CA OUT

) CA

CA - ATPASE

CA

3 NA

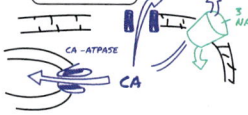

CA = CONTRACTION

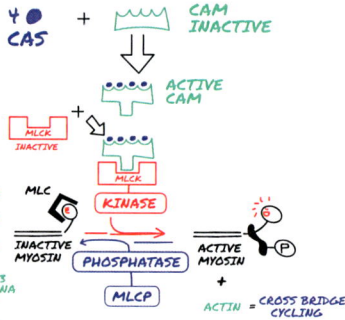

4 CAS + CAM INACTIVE

⬇

ACTIVE CAM

+

MLCK INACTIVE

MLCK

KINASE

MLC

INACTIVE MYOSIN → ACTIVE MYOSIN - P

PHOSPHATASE

MLCP

+

ACTIN = CROSS BRIDGE CYCLING

ANATOMY

- SMALL, FUSIFORM, MONONUCLEAR
- GAP JUNCTIONS = SYNCYTIUM
- DESMOSOMES = HOLD TOGETHER
- DENSE BODIES = "Z LINE" "AROUND"

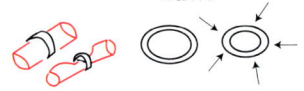

- NO TROPONIN
- 2 MYOSIN HEAVY, 4 LIGHT

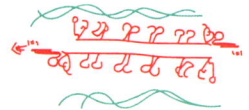

N O T E S

General Physiology

IONIZED

VASCULAR

ABSORBED

$$D = \frac{K \times [GRAD] \times SA}{T \times SIZE}$$

UNIONIZED

K = SOLUBILITY = IONIZED = CLEARED

T   X   SIZE — FREE, UNBOUND

MEMBRANE

$9\ NH_3^+ \rightleftharpoons NH_2 + H^+$

7.4

$2\ COOH \rightleftharpoons COO^- + H^+$

%
IONIZED

PH<PK   PH=PK   PH>PK

PH OF SOLUTION
PH OF DRUG

KINETICS

GEN PRINC
ABSORPTION
DISTRIBUTION
METABOLISM
ELIMINATION

TRANSPORT	[GRAD]	ENERGY	CARRIER	SATURATE	
PASSIVE	↓	= ∅	∅	= ∅	DYNAMICS
FACILITATED	↓	= ∅	⊕	= SATURATION	RECEPTORS
ACTIVE	⬆	= ⊕	⊕	= SATURATION	ANS-SNS PNS CHOLINERGIC ADRENERGICS

NA

K   ATP

Absorption

[PLASMA]

DURATION OF ACTION

CMAX

MEC

O   LAG   TMAX   TIME

ABSORPTION   ELIMINATION
MORE IN THAN OUT   MORE OUT THAN IN

$$D = \frac{K \times [GRAD] \times SA}{T \times SIZE}$$ K=IONIZATION

[PLASMA] 100% IV

BIOAVAILABILITY

$\dfrac{AUC_{IV}}{AUC_{PO}}$

T

PO

MOUTH

PH: 1

PK 9 $NH_3^+ \rightleftharpoons NH_2 + H^+$
PK 2 $COOH \rightleftharpoons COO^- + H^+$

WEAK ACID

IM   SUBQ

WEAK

PH: 10   OUT

SL   TOPICAL
          TD

LIVER

VEINS
IV

L

R

INH

* 1ST-PASS METABOLISM

100%

80% GI

20%   VEINS
1ST-PASS

PR

ROUTE	BARRIER	1ST	BIO
INH	⌣	∅	⌣
IV	∅	∅	100%
IM	↓	∅	90%
SL	↓↓	∅	
SQ	↓↓	∅	
PR	↓↓	∅	>50%
PO	↓↓↓	↓↓	20%
INH	⊘	∅	—

General Pharmacology

Distribution

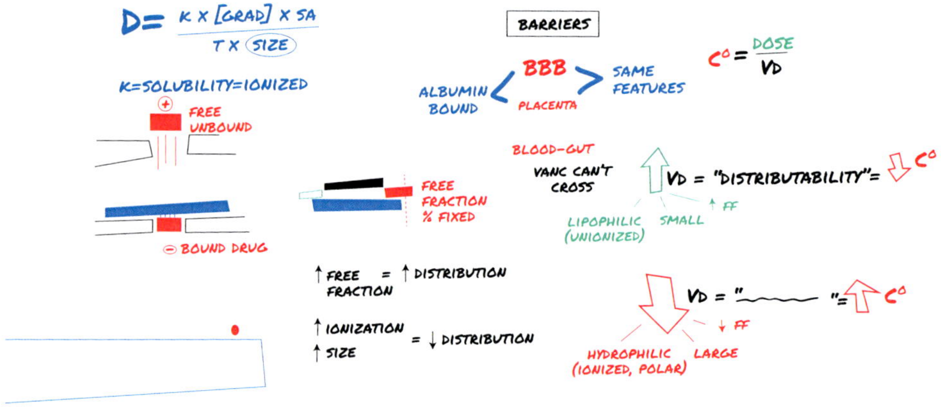

$$D = \frac{K \times [GRAD] \times SA}{T \times \boxed{SIZE}}$$

K = SOLUBILITY = IONIZED

FREE UNBOUND ⊕

⊖ BOUND DRUG

FREE FRACTION % FIXED

↑ FREE FRACTION = ↑ DISTRIBUTION

↑ IONIZATION ↑ SIZE = ↓ DISTRIBUTION

BARRIERS

ALBUMIN BOUND → **BBB** > SAME FEATURES
PLACENTA

BLOOD-GUT
VANC CAN'T CROSS

$$C^0 = \frac{DOSE}{VD}$$

VD = "DISTRIBUTABILITY" = ↓ C^0
LIPOPHILIC (UNIONIZED) SMALL   ↑ FF

VD = "﹏﹏﹏" = ↑ C^0
HYDROPHILIC (IONIZED, POLAR) LARGE   ↓ FF

Metabolism-Biotransformation

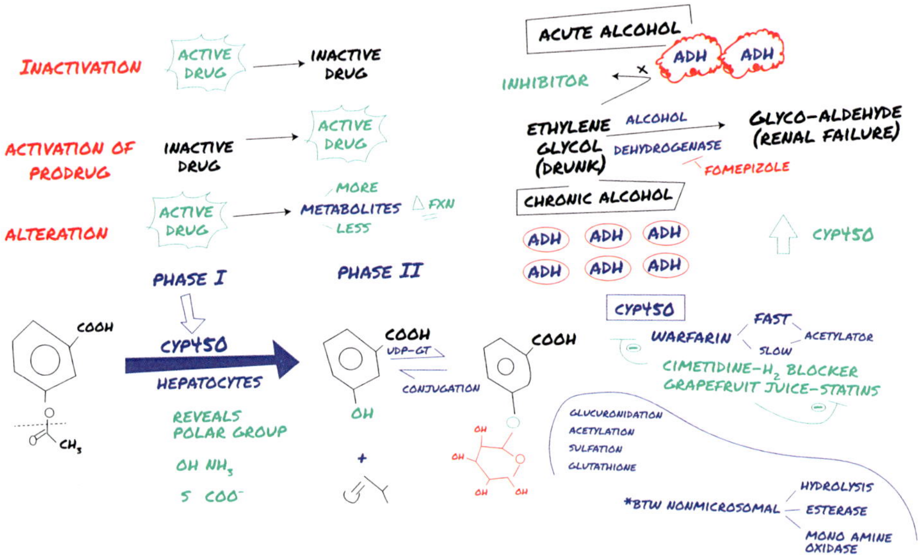

INACTIVATION   ACTIVE DRUG → INACTIVE DRUG

ACTIVATION OF PRODRUG   INACTIVE DRUG → ACTIVE DRUG

ALTERATION   ACTIVE DRUG → MORE METABOLITES LESS △ FXN

PHASE I
⇩
CYP450
HEPATOCYTES
REVEALS POLAR GROUP
OH NH₃
S COO⁻

COOH

PHASE II
COOH
UDP-GT
⇦ CONJUGATION
OH
+

ACUTE ALCOHOL
INHIBITOR ← ✕ ADH ADH

ETHYLENE GLYCOL (DRUNK) ALCOHOL DEHYDROGENASE → GLYCO-ALDEHYDE (RENAL FAILURE)
FOMEPIZOLE

CHRONIC ALCOHOL
ADH ADH ADH
ADH ADH ADH
⇧ CYP450

CYP450
WARFARIN   FAST ACETYLATOR   SLOW
CIMETIDINE-H₂ BLOCKER
GRAPEFRUIT JUICE-STATINS

GLUCURONIDATION
ACETYLATION
SULFATION
GLUTATHIONE

*BTW NONMICROSOMAL — HYDROLYSIS
ESTERASE
MONO AMINE OXIDASE

NOTES

General Pharmacology

Elimination

FILTRATION

SECRETED

ABSORB

CL

RENAL REMOVAL= FILTRATION − ABSORB + SECRETED
DRUG

$CL_{THEORY} = \%FF \times GFR$

$CL_{MEASURE} < CL_{THEORETICAL} = ABSORBED$

$CL_{MEASURE} > CL_{THEORY} = SECRETED$

$$Cl = VD \times K$$

ZERO-ORDER
SATURATED
AMT/TIME (2O)
HALF-LIFE (VAR)
$80 \xrightarrow{2O} 60 \xrightarrow{2O}_{2} 40 \xrightarrow{2O}_{1} 20$

DOSE

LOG

ETOH POISONING

1ST-ORDER
AMT/TIME (VAR)
HALF-LIFE (1)
$80 \xrightarrow{} 40 \xrightarrow{}_{40} 20 \xrightarrow{1}_{20} 10_{10}$

DOSE

LOG

4-7 HALF-LIVES

$$T1/2 = \frac{0.7}{K}$$

$$C^0 = \frac{DOSE}{VD}$$

LOADING DOSE

4-7 HALF-LIVES
MORE TIME
WITHIN THE RANGE
FASTER

DISTRIBUTION
SS
ABSORPTION

$$CL = \frac{VD \times 0.7}{T1/2}$$

ACTIVITY METABOLISM

ELIMINATION

Pharmacodynamics

① PHYSIOLOGIC   SNS   PNS

DRUG %FF

*COMPLETE AGONIST
B $VMAX = VMAX$ C

50%   A

$VMAX = VMAX$ D   CANT

[A] [B] [C] LOG DOSE

X-AXIS = ↑ AFFINITY

Y-AXIS = ↑ EFFICACY # SITES

COMPARISON @ EFF % = ↑ POTENCY

50%   80%
A>B>C B ✶ ✶

② CHEMICAL IVIG ANTIVENOM

DRUG   A

⊕△ Y-AXIS= ↓ #SITES
Ø△ X-AXIS= ⊕△ AFF
NONCOMPETITIVE   B

C

← X-AXIS
↑ AFF
Ø△ # SITES
Ø△ Y-AXIS
POTENTIATOR

⇒ X-AXIS
↓ AFF
Ø△ # SITES
Ø△ Y-AXIS
COMPETITIVE INHIBITOR

100% COMPLETE AGON   PARTIAL AGON   Ø

③ PHARMACOLOGIC

POP

THERAPEUTIC WINDOW   TOXIC WINDOW

% POP

☐ ED50   ☐ TD50
LD50   [DRUG]

$$TI = \frac{TD50}{ED50} \quad OR \quad \frac{LD50}{ED50}$$

OTC 100
RX 10-90
CHEMO 5
DIGOXI 1

General Pharmacology

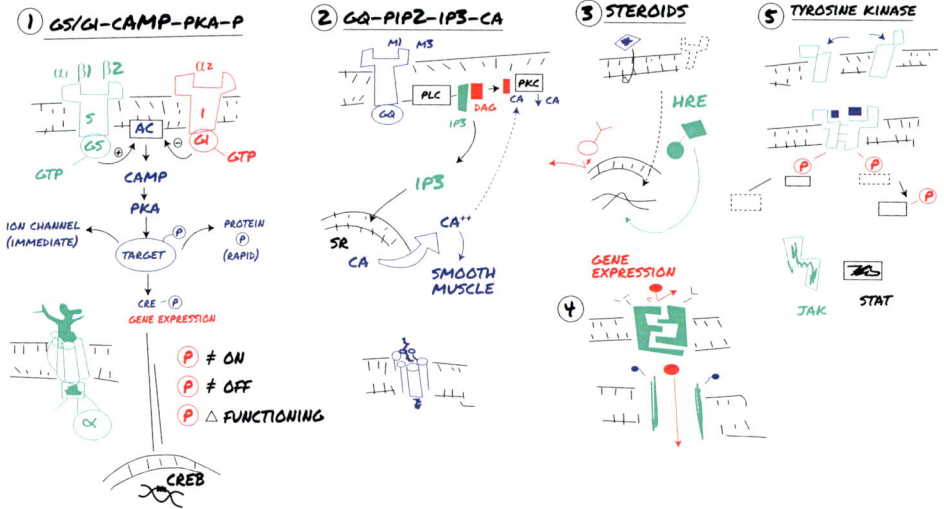

① GS/GI—CAMP—PKA—P

(α) (β) β2 ... (α2)
S
GS — AC — GI
GTP ⊕ ⊖ GTP

CAMP
PKA

ION CHANNEL (IMMEDIATE) → TARGET → (P) → PROTEIN (P) (RAPID)

CRE — (P)
GENE EXPRESSION

(P) ≠ ON
(P) ≠ OFF
(P) △ FUNCTIONING

CREB

α

② GQ—PIP2—IP3—CA

M1 M3
PLC — PKC
GQ — DAG — CA ↓ CA
IP3

IP3
SR
CA
CA⁺⁺
SMOOTH MUSCLE

③ STEROIDS

HRE

GENE EXPRESSION

④

⑤ TYROSINE KINASE

(P) (P) (P)

JAK   STAT

Intro to Autonomics

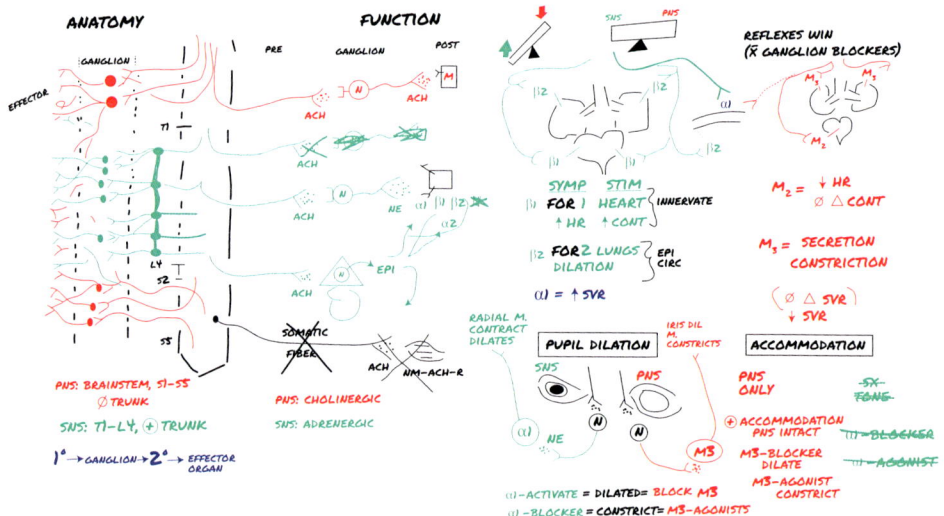

ANATOMY   **FUNCTION**

GANGLION   PRE   GANGLION   POST
EFFECTOR
T1   N   ACH   M
ACH
ACH
N   NE   β1 β2
ACH   α2
L4
S2   N   EPI
ACH
SS
SOMATIC FIBER   ACH   NM—ACH—R

PNS: BRAINSTEM, S1—S5
∅ TRUNK
SNS: T1—L4, ⊕ TRUNK
1° → GANGLION → 2° → EFFECTOR ORGAN

PNS: CHOLINERGIC
SNS: ADRENERGIC

SNS   PNS

REFLEXES WIN
(x̄ GANGLION BLOCKERS)
M2   M2
M2

M2 = ↓ HR
∅ △ CONT
M3 = SECRETION
CONSTRICTION
(∅ △ SVR
↓ SVR)

β1 β2   β2
α

SYMP STIM
β1 FOR ↑ HEART { INNERVATE
↑ HR ↑ CONT
β2 FOR 2 LUNGS { EPI
DILATION   CIRC
α = ↑ SVR

RADIAL M. CONTRACT DILATES
PUPIL DILATION
SNS
α   NE
IRIS DIL M. CONSTRICTS
PNS
N   N   M3

ACCOMMODATION
PNS ONLY   ~~SX TONE~~
⊕ ACCOMMODATION PNS INTACT   ~~M3 BLOCKER~~
M3—BLOCKER DILATE   ~~M3 AGONIST~~
M3—AGONIST CONSTRICT

α—ACTIVATE = DILATED = BLOCK M3
α—BLOCKER = CONSTRICT = M3—AGONISTS

NOTES

Cholinergics (PNS)

① UPTAKE — HEMICHOLINIUM

CHOLINE

CHOLINE + ACETYL-COA

⑧ RENEW

② REFORMATION

ACH

③ VESICLE — EL

CA+

④ DEPOL

⑤ FUSION — BOTULINUM

ACH-ESTERASE

[ACH]

⑦ DEGRADATION

ACH-E-I

MG

[ACH]

⑥ ACTIVITY

NA⁺ K⁺ N M (2ND)

SVR	SYMP	↓ BP
SWEAT	SYMP	↓ SWEAT
HEART	PARA	↑ HR
EYES	PARA	DILATE
GI/GU	PARA	↓ TONE

MEDULLA

N — GANGLION

Nₘ = SKELETAL M.

M₁ EXCROCINE SECRETION GQ-IP3-CA

M₂ NODE ❤ ↓ HR GI-↓ CAMP ↑PKA

M₃ SLUDGE S.M. GQ-IP3-CA²⁺ BRONCHOCONSTRICT

CONTRACTION → CONSTRICTING PUPIL *LES*

M₃ VASODILATION ENDO NO

DIRECT ACTING M-AGONISTS   REVERS + COMP

BETHANECHOL=NEUROGENIC BLADDER
METHACHOLINE (INH) DX ASTHMA
PILOCARPINE (EYE GTT) GLAUCOMA=CONSTRICT

INDIRECT ACTING M-AGONISTS   ACH-E-I

                        → MG
(LIPID) PHYSIO ⎤
NEO   ⎥—STIGMINE   PERIPHERAL.....OGILVIE
PYRIDO ⎦
EDROPHONIUM   DX MG, TOO SHORT ACTING
(LIPID) ORGANOPHOSPHATES PESTICIDES, NERVE GAS
                ↓ AGING: PRALIDOXIME
                "AGE" ACH-E
                ATROPINE= ↓ SXS

REVERS

Irr

MUSCARINIC ANTAGONISTS

ATROPINE (IV) ORGANOPHOSPHATE, BRADY
IPRATROPIUM (INH), OLD (COPD/ASTHMA)
SCOPOLAMINE (TD), N/V, "MOTION SICKNESS"

NICOTINIC ANTAGONISTS   *NEVER USED*

HEXAMETHONIUM ⎤ GANGLIONIC
MECAMYLAMINE ⎦ BLOCK

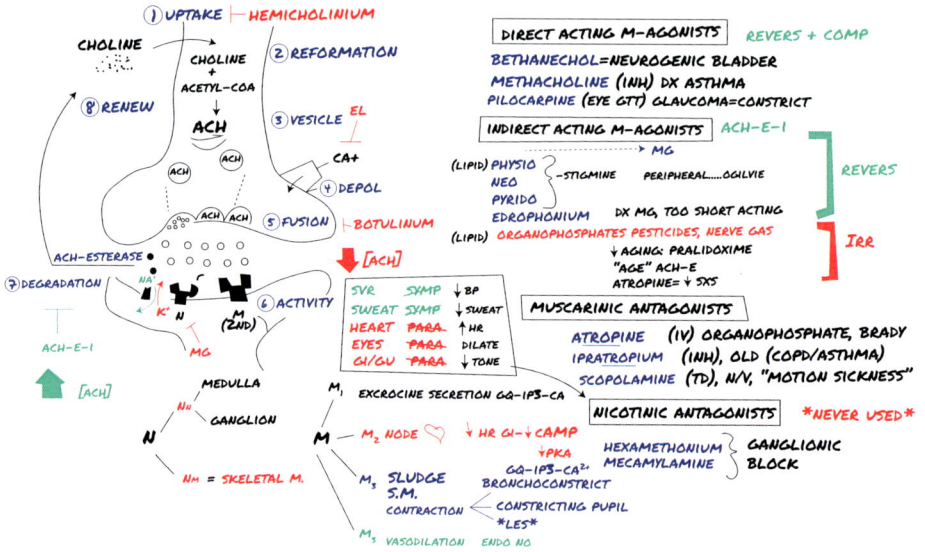

Adrenergics (SNS)

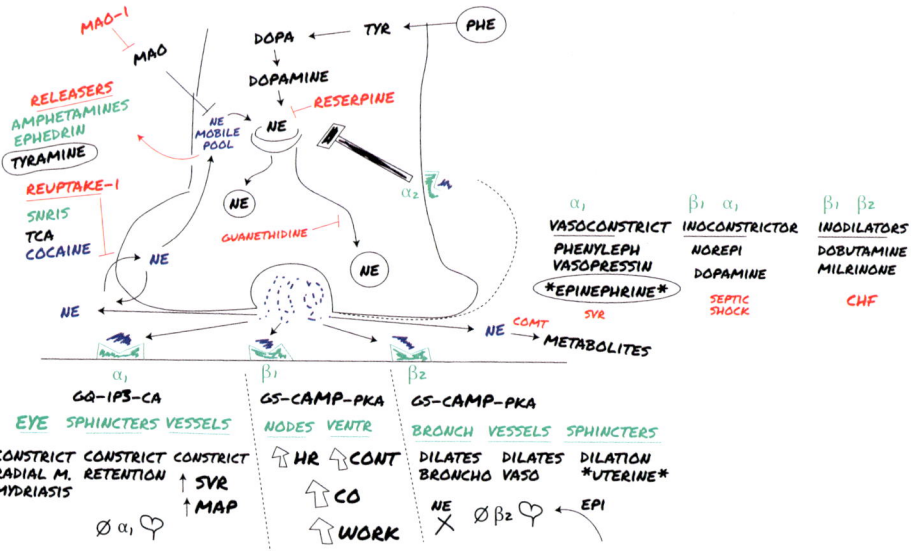

MAO-I
MAO

RELEASERS
AMPHETAMINES
EPHEDRIN
TYRAMINE

REUPTAKE-I
SNRIS
TCA
COCAINE

PHE → TYR → DOPA
DOPAMINE
NE MOBILE POOL — RESERPINE
NE

NE

GUANETHIDINE

NE

α₂

NE

NE

NE COMT
→ METABOLITES

α₁	β₁ α₁	β₁ β₂
VASOCONSTRICT	INOCONSTRICTOR	INODILATORS
PHENYLEPH	NOREPI	DOBUTAMINE
VASOPRESSIN	DOPAMINE	MILRINONE
EPINEPHRINE	SEPTIC SHOCK	CHF
SVR		

α₁	β₁	β₂
GQ-IP3-CA	GS-CAMP-PKA	GS-CAMP-PKA
EYE SPHINCTERS VESSELS	NODES VENTR	BRONCH VESSELS SPHINCTERS
CONSTRICT CONSTRICT CONSTRICT	↑HR ↑CONT	DILATES DILATES DILATION
RADIAL M. RETENTION	⬆ CO	BRONCHO VASO *UTERINE*
MYDRIASIS	⬆ WORK	
∅ α₁ ❤	↑SVR ↑MAP	NE ✗ ∅ β₂ ❤ — EPI

NOTES

General Pharmacology

Cellular Adaptations

OnlineMedEd

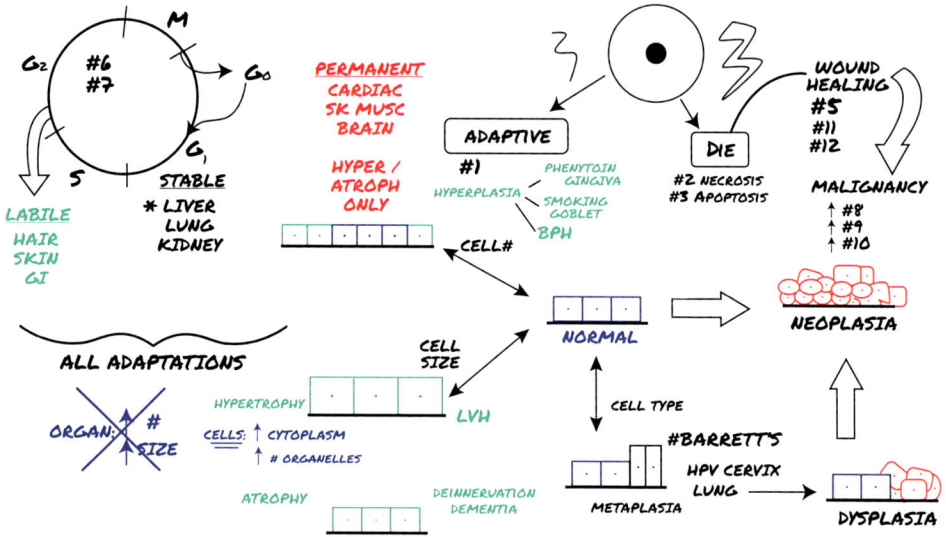

Cell cycle diagram:
G₂ — #6 #7 — M — G₀
S, G₁
STABLE
* LIVER LUNG KIDNEY

LABILE
HAIR SKIN GI

PERMANENT
CARDIAC
SK MUSC
BRAIN

HYPER / ATROPH ONLY

ADAPTIVE #1
HYPERPLASIA — PHENYTOIN GINGIVA, SMOKING GOBLET, BPH

CELL #

DIE
#2 NECROSIS
#3 APOPTOSIS

WOUND HEALING
#5 #11 #12

MALIGNANCY
↑ #8
↑ #9
↑ #10

NORMAL → NEOPLASIA

CELL SIZE

ALL ADAPTATIONS

ORGAN: ↑ # ↑ SIZE

HYPERTROPHY
CELLS: ↑ CYTOPLASM
↑ # ORGANELLES

ATROPHY
DEINNERVATION
DEMENTIA

LVH

CELL TYPE

#BARRETT'S
HPV CERVIX
LUNG

METAPLASIA

DYSPLASIA

Necrosis

NECROSIS:
- UNPROGRAMMED
- DEATH, FRAGMENTATION
- SWELLING → LYSIS
- ⊕ INFLAMMATION
- ∅ MEMBRANE-BOUND
- MANY CELLS AFFECTED

APOPTOSIS
- PROGRAMMED, SEQUENCE
- ORGANIZED DISASSEMBLY
- MEMBRANE-BOUND
- SHRINKS, ∅ INFLAMMATION
- ONE CELL, SMALL CLUSTERS

EARLY: ORGANELLES (SER, MITO) REVER
LATE: CELL MEMBRANE REVERS NUCLEUS...BLEBBING
IRR: PERFORATION = LYSIS
CA^{++} INFLUX = MITO BODIES

TYPE / CAUSED BY
COAGULATIVE — ISCHEMIA INFARCT — ① ↓ ATP
DRY →

LIQUEFACTIVE — CNS INFARCTS (AUTOLYSIS)
WET ⇨ PYOGENIC INFXN (HETEROLYSIS)

CASEOUS — TB (99%) ⇨ AFB, FUNGI

FAT — ENZYMATIC = LIPASE / PANCREATITIS
NONENZYMATIC = TRAUMATIC

FIBRINOID — VASCULITIS

PATHOGENESIS
TCA ETC ATP
GLUCOSE → LACTATE
② ↓ PH
PYRUVATE
O₂
−O₂

① ↓ ATP = NA/K ATPASE (WATER, IONS) SWELLS
② ↓ PH = DENATURATION

∅ GLYCOGEN = ∅ GLUCOSE + ∅ O₂ = ∅ DENATURE
↓ ATP = SWELL + LYSIS
PMN, BACTERIA = DIGESTIVE

"WALLING OFF" BY MACROPHAGES
⊕ MULTINUCLEATED GIANT CELLS

C C C → HYDROLYSIS → C C C + ξξξ
ξ + SALT = SOAP CA^{++}
TYPE IV

HISTO / PATH
⊕ CELL ARCHITECTURE
⇧ PINK
∅ NUCLEUS
PALE + FIRM / RED + FIRM
SOUP

"MOTH-EATEN" VACUOLES

SHEETS OF PINK SURROUNDED BY BLUE CELLS
GRANULOMA

SAPONIFICATION
ADIPOSE : CHALKY WHITE
ADIPOSE : CHUNKS
SAPONIFICATION

80

© 2020 OnlineMedEd

Inflammation and Neoplasia

Apoptosis

FAILED TROPHIC = INTRINSIC

CASPASE
INITIATOR EFFECTOR
8, 9 3

AKT

INTRINSIC

EXTRINSIC = DEATH-R

FAS-FASL   TNF-α   PERFORINS

BAX (PRO)   BCL-2 (ANTI)

ANT

CYTC

BAD (PRO)   BAD

BAX:BAX

TRIMER

L R

FADD

CYT C

BID

GRANZYME B

BAX : BCL-2

BAD:BCL2   BAX:BAX

NOVA PUMA

(APAF1), CAS9)

LOW AFF

MDM

P

SENESCENCE

DMG DNA   ↑P53   ↑BAX   BAX: BAX
INTRINSIC   ↓BCL-2

DMG DNA = INTRINSIC

P

HIGH AFF
ARREST CELL CYCLE
DNA REPAIR

FAILURE OF   ↓AKT   ↑BAD   BAX: BAX
TROPH   ↓BCL-2

ATM   ATM   KINASE

ATM
DMG DNA

ATM   CHK2   KINASE   MDM

EXTRINSIC   DEATH-R   8
                      PC3 → 3

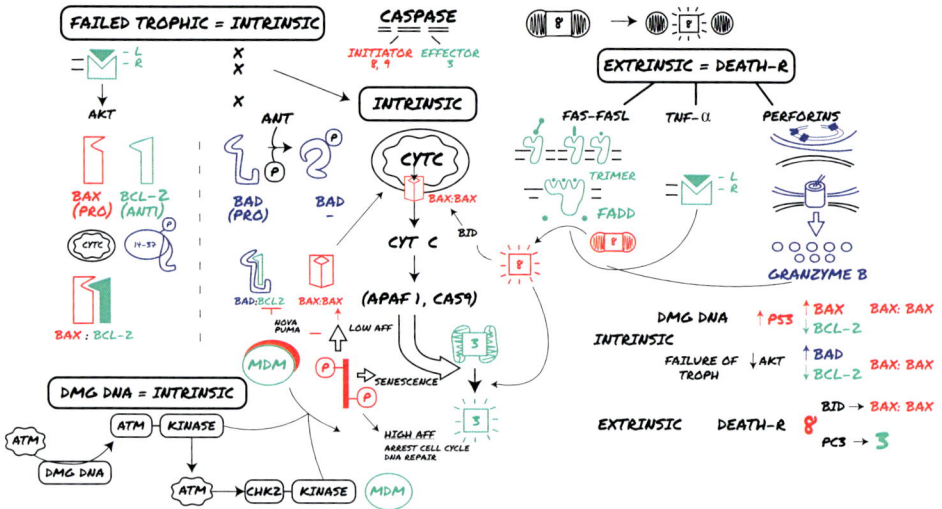

Wound Healing

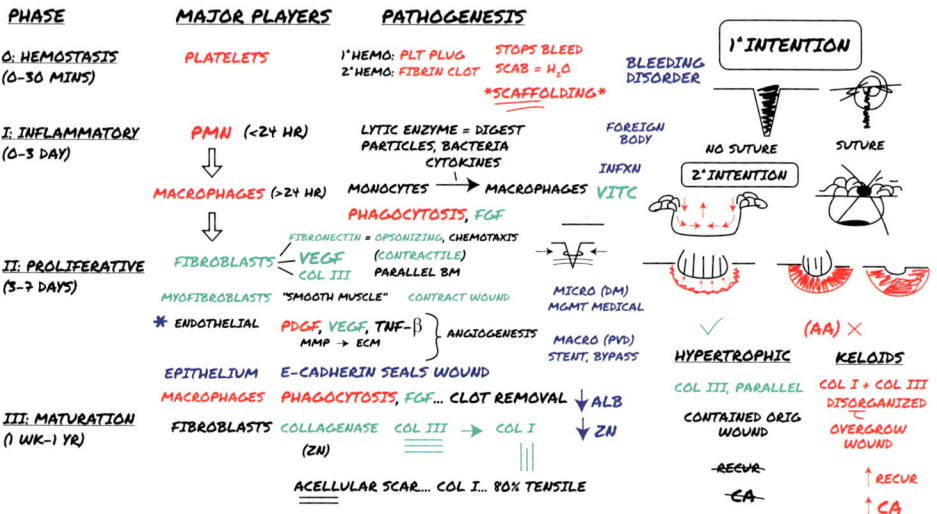

PHASE	MAJOR PLAYERS	PATHOGENESIS

0: HEMOSTASIS (0-30 MINS)   PLATELETS   1°HEMO: PLT PLUG   2°HEMO: FIBRIN CLOT   STOPS BLEED   SCAB = H₂O   *SCAFFOLDING*

BLEEDING DISORDER

1°INTENTION

NO SUTURE   SUTURE

I: INFLAMMATORY (0-3 DAY)   PMN (<24 HR)   LYTIC ENZYME = DIGEST PARTICLES, BACTERIA   CYTOKINES   FOREIGN BODY   INFXN   VITC

MACROPHAGES (>24 HR)   MONOCYTES → MACROPHAGES
PHAGOCYTOSIS, FGF

2°INTENTION

II: PROLIFERATIVE (3-7 DAYS)   FIBROBLASTS   FIBRONECTIN = OPSONIZING, CHEMOTAXIS   VEGF (CONTRACTILE)   COL III   PARALLEL BM
MYOFIBROBLASTS "SMOOTH MUSCLE" CONTRACT WOUND   MICRO (DM) MGMT MEDICAL
* ENDOTHELIAL   PDGF, VEGF, TNF-β   MMP → ECM   ANGIOGENESIS   MACRO (PVD) STENT, BYPASS
EPITHELIUM   E-CADHERIN SEALS WOUND
MACROPHAGES   PHAGOCYTOSIS, FGF... CLOT REMOVAL   ↓ALB   ↓ZN

HYPERTROPHIC   (AA) ×   KELOIDS
COL III, PARALLEL   COL I + COL III DISORGANIZED
CONTAINED ORIG WOUND   OVERGROW WOUND
RECUR   ↑RECUR
CA   ↑CA

III: MATURATION (1 WK-1 YR)   FIBROBLASTS   COLLAGENASE   COL III → COL I   (ZN)

ACELLULAR SCAR... COL I... 80% TENSILE

NOTES

G_2

↑ CYTOPLASM
ORGANELLES

M

P
PM
M
A
CYTO

CELL IS ITSELF

G_0

GROWTH FACTORS

DECISIONS (REGULATION)

DNA CHECKS

REPLICATION

G_1

XX

4N

S PHASE REPLICATE

2N

PERMANENT: NEVER ENTER CYCLE
SK MUS, CARD MUS, BRAIN

STABLE G_0 ... INDUCED INTO CYCLE

LABILE: ALWAYS IN CYCLE
GI, SKIN, HAIR, NAILS

G_2

PRO

PM

M   ASTRAL

A

T   ACTIN

C

G_1

LAMIN DEGRADES ENVELOPE
HISTONES H1 CONDENSES DNA
TUBULIN MT, MTOC

MT, TUG-OF-WAR

KINETOCHORE

KINETOCHORE

CENTROMERE REGION

− END

GTP

+ PLUS

− END

KINETOCHORE

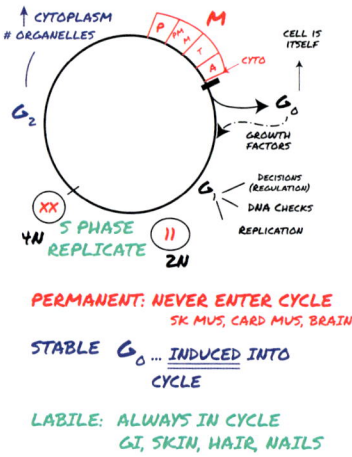

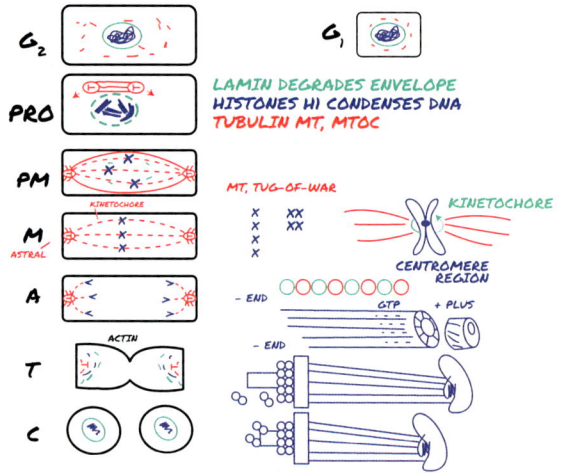

Cell Cycle Regulation

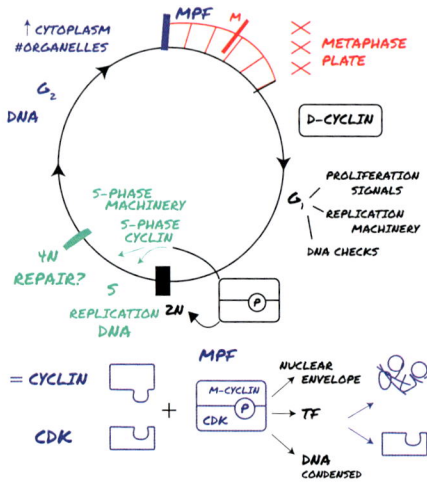

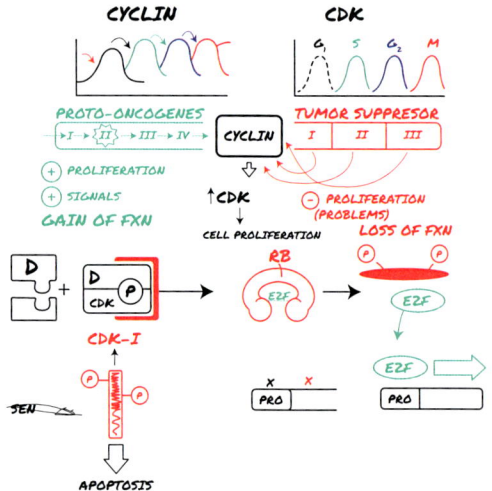

MPF M

↑ CYTOPLASM
#ORGANELLES

G_2
DNA

METAPHASE PLATE

D-CYCLIN

PROLIFERATION SIGNALS

REPLICATION MACHINERY

DNA CHECKS

G_1

S-PHASE MACHINERY
S-PHASE CYCLIN

4N
REPAIR?

S

REPLICATION 2N
DNA

P

= CYCLIN

CDK

MPF

M-CYCLIN
CDK
P

NUCLEAR ENVELOPE

TF

DNA CONDENSED

CYCLIN

CDK

G_1 S G_2 M

PROTO-ONCOGENES

I → II → III → IV

CYCLIN

(+) PROLIFERATION
(+) SIGNALS
GAIN OF FXN

↑CDK

CELL PROLIFERATION

TUMOR SUPPRESOR

I	II	III

(−) PROLIFERATION (PROBLEMS)

LOSS OF FXN

D + D
        CDK P

CDK-I

P

P

SEN

APOPTOSIS

RB

E2F

E2F

x   x
PRO

P   P

E2F

E2F

PRO

Biology of Cancer

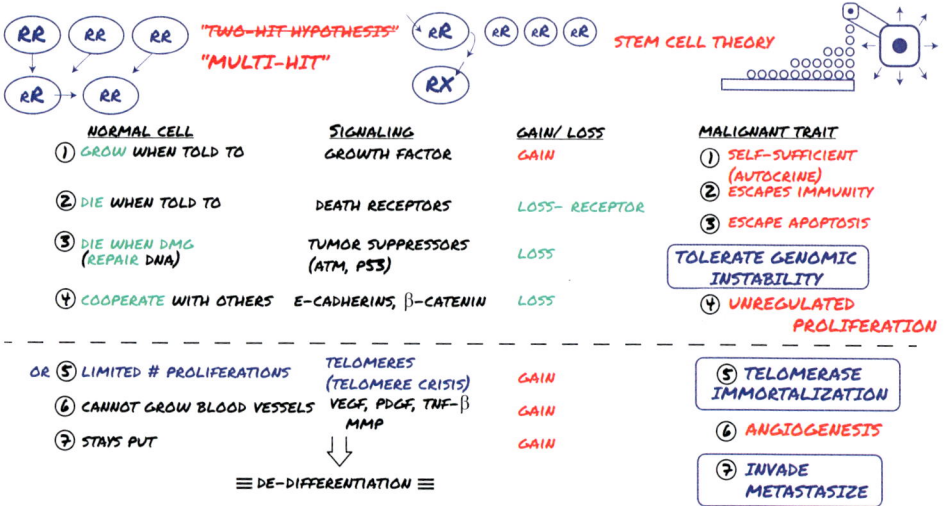

"TWO-HIT HYPOTHESIS"
"MULTI-HIT"

STEM CELL THEORY

NORMAL CELL	SIGNALING	GAIN/ LOSS	MALIGNANT TRAIT
① GROW WHEN TOLD TO	GROWTH FACTOR	GAIN	① SELF-SUFFICIENT (AUTOCRINE)
② DIE WHEN TOLD TO	DEATH RECEPTORS	LOSS- RECEPTOR	② ESCAPES IMMUNITY
③ DIE WHEN DMG (REPAIR DNA)	TUMOR SUPPRESSORS (ATM, P53)	LOSS	③ ESCAPE APOPTOSIS
			TOLERATE GENOMIC INSTABILITY
④ COOPERATE WITH OTHERS	E-CADHERINS, β-CATENIN	LOSS	④ UNREGULATED PROLIFERATION

OR ⑤ LIMITED # PROLIFERATIONS — TELOMERES (TELOMERE CRISIS) — GAIN — ⑤ TELOMERASE IMMORTALIZATION

⑥ CANNOT GROW BLOOD VESSELS — VEGF, PDGF, TNF-β MMP — GAIN — ⑥ ANGIOGENESIS

⑦ STAYS PUT — GAIN — ⑦ INVADE METASTASIZE

≡ DE-DIFFERENTIATION ≡

Cell Cycle Chemotherapy

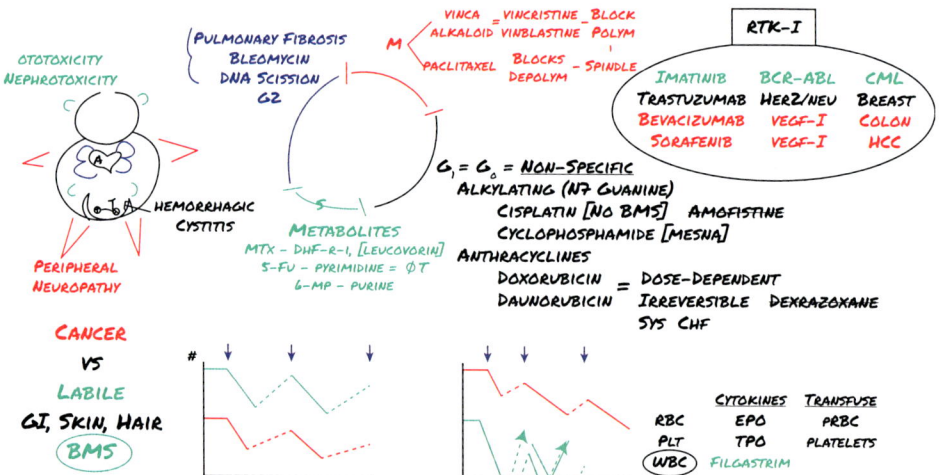

OTOTOXICITY
NEPHROTOXICITY

PULMONARY FIBROSIS
BLEOMYCIN
DNA SCISSION
G2

VINCA = VINCRISTINE _ BLOCK
ALKALOID VINBLASTINE POLYM
PACLITAXEL _ BLOCKS
DEPOLYM — SPINDLE

RTK-I

IMATINIB	BCR-ABL	CML
TRASTUZUMAB	HER2/NEU	BREAST
BEVACIZUMAB	VEGF-I	COLON
SORAFENIB	VEGF-I	HCC

$G_1 = G_0 =$ NON-SPECIFIC

ALKYLATING (N7 GUANINE)
CISPLATIN [NO BMS] AMOFISTINE
CYCLOPHOSPHAMIDE [MESNA]

ANTHRACYCLINES
DOXORUBICIN = DOSE-DEPENDENT
DAUNORUBICIN = IRREVERSIBLE DEXRAZOXANE
SYS CHF

HEMORRHAGIC CYSTITIS

METABOLITES
MTX - DHF-R-I, [LEUCOVORIN]
5-FU - PYRIMIDINE = Ø T
6-MP - PURINE

PERIPHERAL NEUROPATHY

CANCER
VS
LABILE
GI, SKIN, HAIR
BMS

	CYTOKINES	TRANSFUSE
RBC	EPO	PRBC
PLT	TPO	PLATELETS
WBC	FILGASTRIM	

Inflammation and Neoplasia

Epidemiology of Cancer

MORTALITY

♂ = ♀

650K 1. CAD/CHF
600K 2. CANCER
⋮
150K 3. LUNG DZ (COPD)
140K 4. CVA
110K 5. AD

CA INCIDENCE

♂
SKIN
[PROSTATE]
LUNG
COLON

♀
SKIN
[BREAST]
LUNG
COLON

CA MORTALITY

♂
LUNG
[PROSTATE] ≈
COLON
PANCREAS

♀
LUNG
[BREAST]
COLON
PANCREAS

NET
LUNG
BREAST
PROSTATE
COLON
PANCREAS

VIRUSES + CANCER

HPV   CERVICAL/ANAL   VACCINATE
EBV   BURKITT'S LYMPHOMA
HEP B   HCC W/O CIRRHOSIS
HEP C   HCC C CIRRHOSIS
HHV-8   KAPOSI'S SARCOMA

METS

1° BRAIN Ø MET
TO BRAIN: LUNG > BREAST > MELANOMA > COLON, RENAL
          WELL-CIRCUMSCRIBED GREY-WHITE, MULTIPLE
TO LIVER: COLON >>> STOMACH, PANCREAS
          PORTAL CIRCULATION
TO BONE: PROSTATE = BREAST >> LUNG/THYROID/RENAL
         (BLASTIC) (MIXED)   (LYTIC)

NAMES

"EPITHELIUM"
CARCINOMA
SQUAMOUS
ADENOCARCINOMA
COLON
BREAST
PROSTATE

BLOOD VESSELS
MUSCLES
JOINTS
BONE
CARTILAGE
SARCOMA
OSTEO - SARCOMA
LEIOMYO - "
RHABDO - "
ANGIO - "
GERMINOMA
DYSGERMINOMA
SEMINOMA

BM...LYMPH
↓
LYMPHOMA
HODGKINS
NON-HODGKINS

BM...BLOOD
↓
LEUKEMIA
AML CML
ALL CLL

SPREAD

LYMPH   HEMA   LOCAL
CARCINOMAS   SARCOMAS   OVARIAN
                               PANCREATIC
  └→ x̄ → RENAL CELL
          HCC
          FOLLICULAR
          CHORI

SCREEN + PREV

CANCER	AGE START	SCREEN	PREV
LUNG	55-85 > 30PY ≤ 15 YRS LAST	LOW DOSE CT Q1Y	SMOKING CESSATION
COLON	50 OR 10 YRS B 1° RELATIVE	COLON Q10Y OR FLEX Q3Y + FOBT Q5Y OR FOBT Q1Y	RED MEAT
BREAST	40 Q1 OR Q2 (50 Q2Y) SBE CBE	MAMMOGRAM MAMMOGRAM	SCREEN
CERVICAL	21 —————— 30 ——————	PAP Q3Y PAP+HPV Q5Y	VACCINE HPV
PROSTATE	DON'T SCREEN PSA+DRE IF AA + 1° DX < 65		
HCC	HEP B, CIRRHOSIS	AFP + U/S Q6M Q12M	ETOH, TREAT C VACCIN B

TEST - TAKING

CLUE	CANCER	MECHANISM
JAPAN	GASTRIC	NITROSAMINES
SE ASIA	HCC	HEP B VERT HORIZ IN HOSP
SHIPYARDS CONSTRUCTION	BRONCHOGENIC LUNG	ASBESTOSIS
PLEURAL PLAQUES	MESOTHELIOMA	
DRY CLEANING	BLADDER	β-ALANINE DYER
RADIOLOGIST	THYROID	NO LEAD
SUN, SAILOR	SKIN	UVB + UVA

General Concepts of Neoplasia

CANCER GROWTH

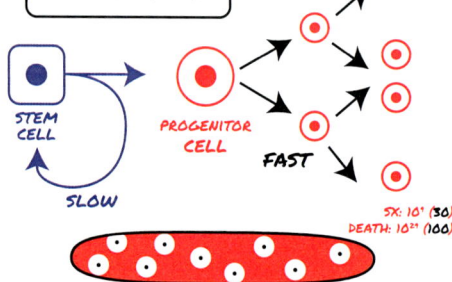

STEM CELL — SLOW → PROGENITOR CELL → FAST
5X: 10^9 (30)
DEATH: 10^{21} (100)

DOUBLING TIME

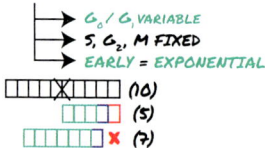

G_0 / G_1 VARIABLE
S, G_2, M FIXED
EARLY = EXPONENTIAL

(10)
(5)
(7)

GROWTH FRACTION % ↑ POP
STAGNATION FRACTION % Ø △ POP
DEATH FRACTION % ↓ POP

CARCINOMA PROGRESSION

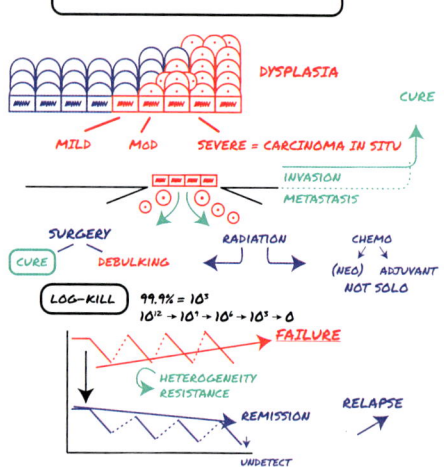

DYSPLASIA
MILD MOD SEVERE = CARCINOMA IN SITU
INVASION
METASTASIS
CURE

SURGERY   RADIATION   CHEMO
CURE DEBULKING   (NEO) ADJUVANT
                        NOT SOLO

LOG-KILL   99.9% = 10^3
$10^{12} → 10^9 → 10^6 → 10^3 → 0$

FAILURE
HETEROGENEITY
RESISTANCE
REMISSION   RELAPSE
UNDETECT

Online MedEd

THE CELLS
DIAGNOSIS

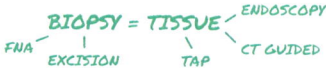

BIOPSY = TISSUE
- ENDOSCOPY
- FNA
- EXCISION
- TAP
- CT GUIDED

GRADE
① (DE) DIFFERENTIATION
② MITOTIC RATE

STAIN
- CONFIRM DX
- EXPRESSING X?

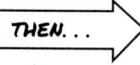

THEN...

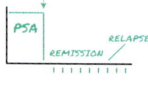

PSA · RELAPSE
REMISSION

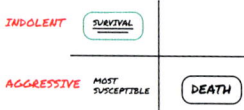

WELL   ANAPLASTIC

INDOLENT — SURVIVAL

AGGRESSIVE — MOST SUSCEPTIBLE — DEATH

BREAST CA — HER2/NEU TRASTUZUMAB
ERP/ PR SERM
AROMATASE-I

CML — T9:22, BCR-ABL — PCR — IMATINIB
JAK-STAT — PHILADELPHIA — FISH

ALL — CD 10 = CALLA
LYMPHOMA — CD 15/30 = HODGKINS
CD 3, 4, 8 = T-CELLS
CD 20 = B-CELLS

THE HUMAN
STAGING

TUMOR SIZE
INVASION — GOOD
NODES
METS — POOR
METS > NODES > TUMOR

I	∅ INVASION – CURE	
II	⊕ INVASION – CURE	
	∅ NODES	↑ REMISSION
III	⊕ INVASION – CURE	
	⊕ NODES	↓ REMISSION
IV	⊕ METS – DEATH	

SCAN

BX — IMAGING = PET(CT)
PAN SCAN

TRACK ≠ DIAGNOSE

AFP : HCC, NON-SEMINOMA
β-HCG : CHORIO TROPHOBLASTIC
CA 19-9 : PANCREATIC   PSA, PROSTATE
CA 125 : OVARIAN
CEA : COLON

Inflammation and Neoplasia

Introduction to Immunology

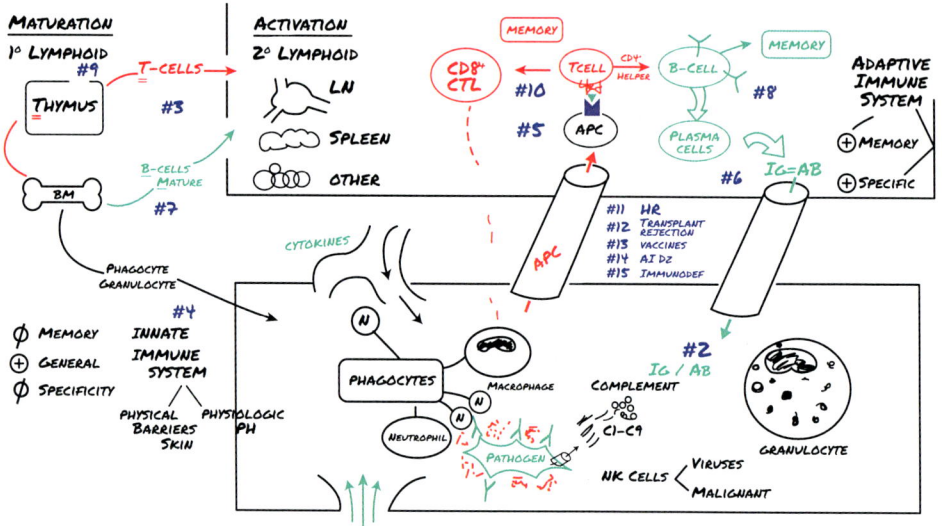

Taxonomy of Immune Cells

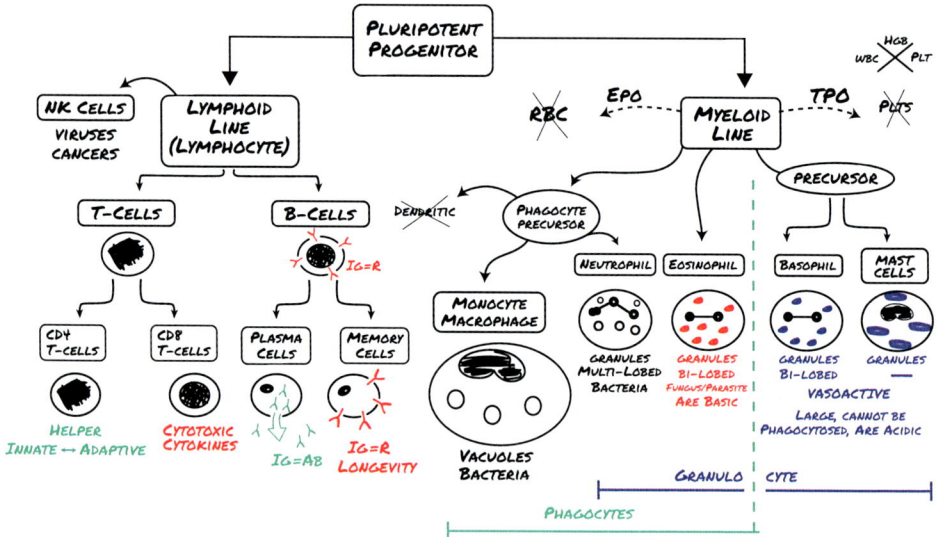

Taxonomy of Lymphoid Organs

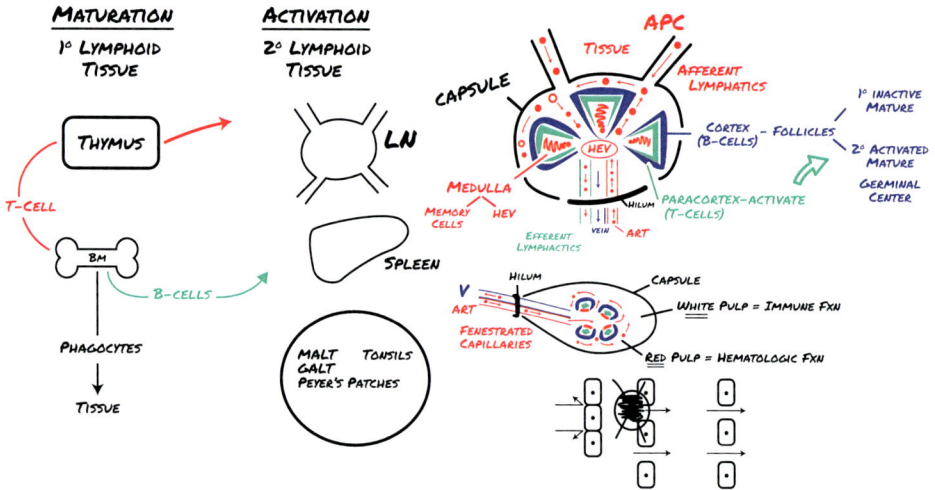

MATURATION
1° LYMPHOID TISSUE

ACTIVATION
2° LYMPHOID TISSUE

THYMUS

T-CELL

BM

B-CELLS

PHAGOCYTES

TISSUE

LN

SPLEEN

MALT   TONSILS
GALT
PEYER'S PATCHES

APC
TISSUE
CAPSULE
AFFERENT LYMPHATICS
CORTEX (B-CELLS) - FOLLICLES
HEV
MEDULLA
MEMORY CELLS   HEV
EFFERENT LYMPHATICS
HILUM   VEIN   ART
PARACORTEX-ACTIVATE (T-CELLS)

1° INACTIVE MATURE
2° ACTIVATED MATURE
GERMINAL CENTER

CAPSULE
V   HILUM
ART
FENESTRATED CAPILLARIES
WHITE PULP = IMMUNE FXN
RED PULP = HEMATOLOGIC FXN

Innate Immune Response

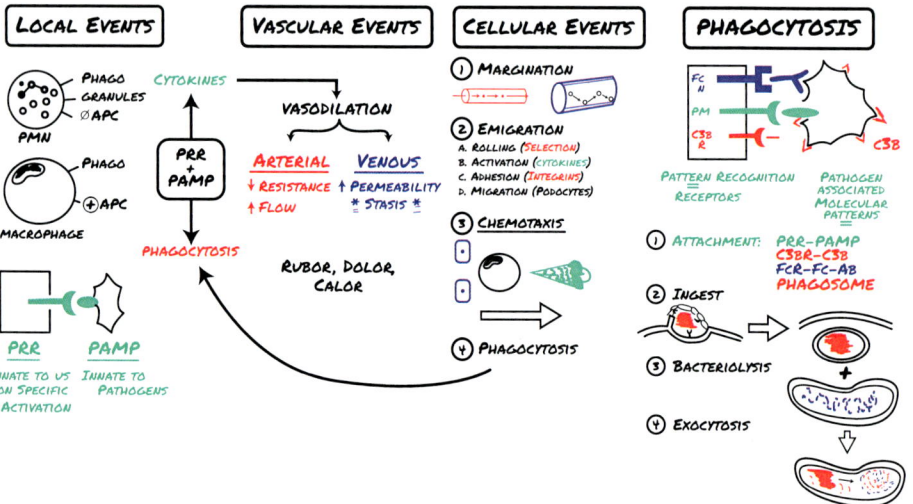

LOCAL EVENTS

PHAGO GRANULES
ØAPC
PMN

PHAGO
⊕APC
MACROPHAGE

PRR + PAMP

CYTOKINES

PHAGOCYTOSIS

PRR
INNATE TO US
NON SPECIFIC
φ ACTIVATION

PAMP
INNATE TO PATHOGENS

VASCULAR EVENTS

VASODILATION

ARTERIAL
↓ RESISTANCE
↑ FLOW

VENOUS
↑ PERMEABILITY
* STASIS *

RUBOR, DOLOR, CALOR

CELLULAR EVENTS

1) MARGINATION

2) EMIGRATION
A. ROLLING (SELECTION)
B. ACTIVATION (CYTOKINES)
C. ADHESION (INTEGRINS)
D. MIGRATION (PODOCYTES)

3) CHEMOTAXIS

4) PHAGOCYTOSIS

PHAGOCYTOSIS

Fc N
PM
C3B R
C3B

PATTERN RECOGNITION RECEPTORS =
PATHOGEN ASSOCIATED MOLECULAR PATTERNS

1) ATTACHMENT: PRR-PAMP
C3BR-C3B
FCR-FC-AB
PHAGOSOME

2) INGEST

3) BACTERIOLYSIS

4) EXOCYTOSIS

Immunology

APCs and MHCs

SELF-AG
CYTOTOXIC CD8 T-CELLS
VIRUS
MALIGNANCY
B-2 MICROGLOBULIN
INDUCE APOPTOSIS
ALL CELLS
FAILURE TO PRESENT AG ⊖

FOREIGN AG
BACTERIA FUNGI ⎤→ ABR → CD4 HELPER
IG → T-CELLS
APC
CLIP, DM
⊕ FINDING

MHC-I
8/MHC=CD8 (I)

MHC-II
8/MHC=CD4 (II)
+DM
-DM
MHC=HLA

GENETIC RESTRICTION
CD8-MHC-AG^x

MHC
NUCLEUS
SELF-AG "SAFEWORD"
MCH II - CLIP

T AG'
AG'
T AG'
AG'

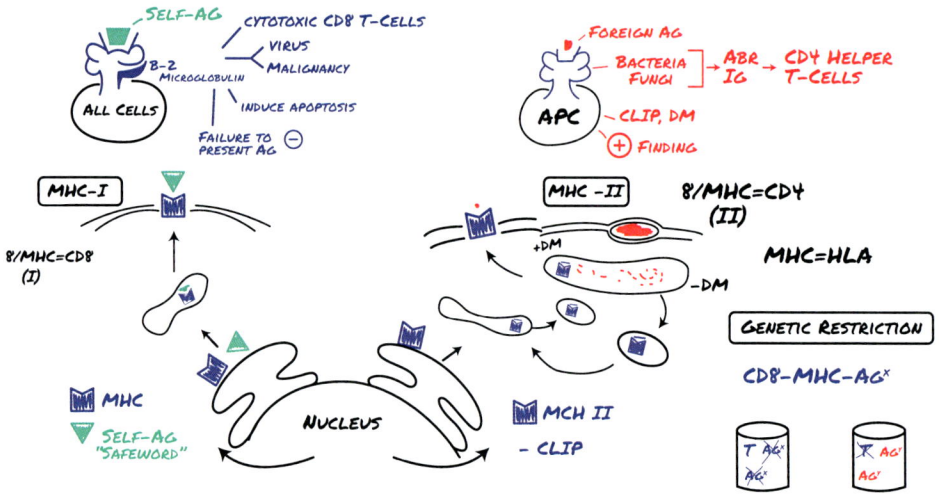

Antigens and Antibodies

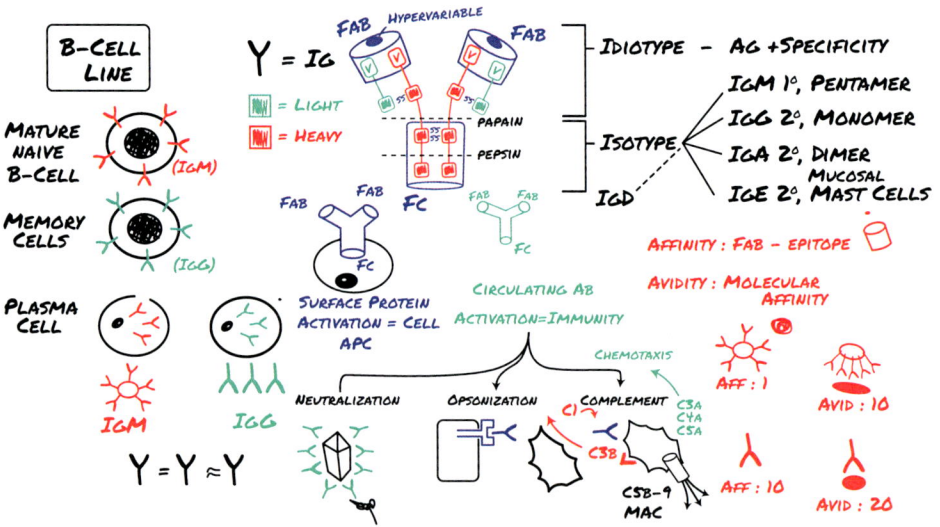

B-CELL LINE

MATURE NAIVE B-CELL (IGM)

MEMORY CELLS (IGG)

PLASMA CELL

IGM   IGG

$Y = Y \approx Y$

$Y = IG$
FAB   HYPERVARIABLE   FAB
= LIGHT
= HEAVY
PAPAIN
PEPSIN
FAB   FAB
FC
FAB   FAB
FC
FC
SURFACE PROTEIN
ACTIVATION = CELL
APC

IDIOTYPE - AG +SPECIFICITY
IGM 1°, PENTAMER
IGG 2°, MONOMER
ISOTYPE
IGA 2°, DIMER MUCOSAL
IGE 2°, MAST CELLS
IGD

AFFINITY: FAB - EPITOPE
AVIDITY: MOLECULAR AFFINITY

CIRCULATING AB
ACTIVATION = IMMUNITY
CHEMOTAXIS
NEUTRALIZATION   OPSONIZATION   COMPLEMENT
C3A C4A C5A
C1
C3B
C5B-9 MAC

AFF: 1
AVID: 10
AFF: 10
AVID: 20

Immunology

B-Cell Maturation

OnlineMedEd

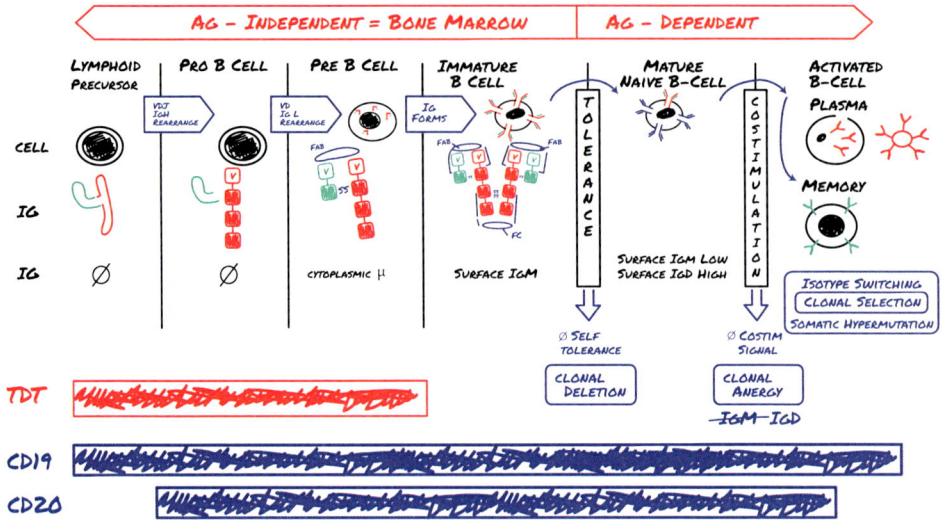

B-Cell Activation

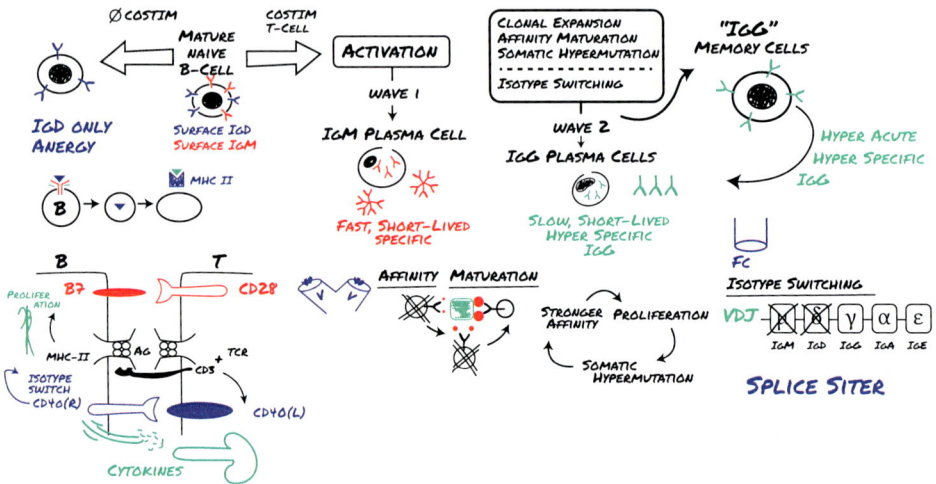

Immunology

T-Cell Maturation

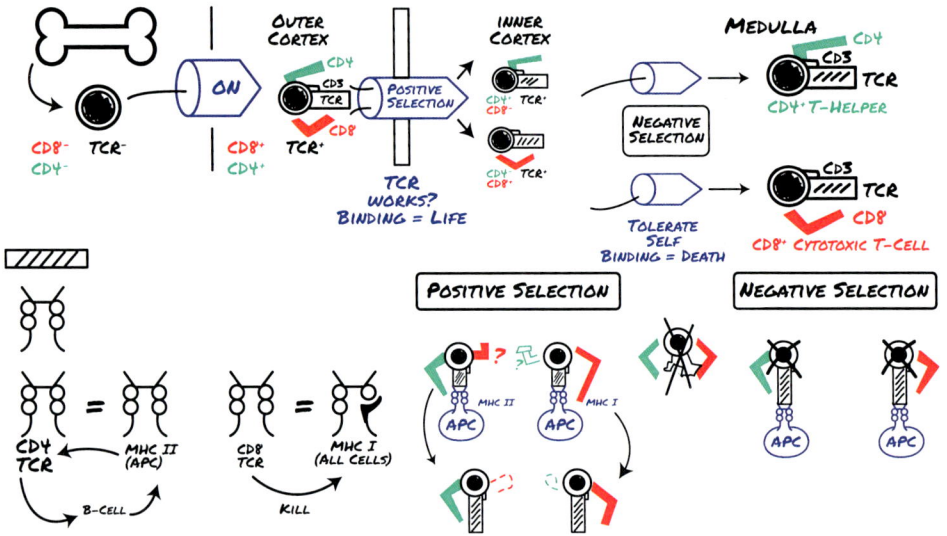

T-Cell Activation

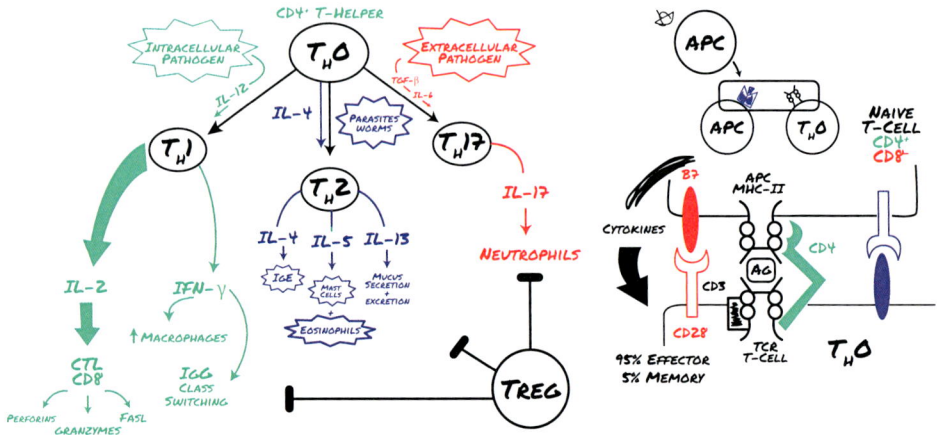

NOTES

Hypersensitivity Reactions

IGE – MAST CELL
1°: SENSITIZATION
2°: IMMEDIATE: DEGRANULATION
LONG-TERM: PROSTAGLANDINS
LEUKOTRIENES

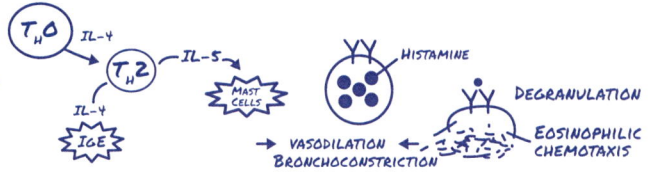

$T_H 0 \rightarrow$ IL-4 $\rightarrow T_H 2 \rightarrow$ IL-5 $\rightarrow$ MAST CELLS

IL-4 → IGE

HISTAMINE
DEGRANULATION
EOSINOPHILIC CHEMOTAXIS
→ VASODILATION ←
BRONCHOCONSTRICTION

CYTOTOXIC-AB OPSONIZATION
Fc-DEPENDENT ← NEUTRALIZATION
COMPLEMENT

NONCYTOTOXIC-AB Ca⁺⁺
Fc-DEPENDENT
AB ↑ OR ↓ FXN

c_i → SELF → PHAGOCYTOSIS
C5-9
EATON-LAMBERT
MYASTHENIA
GRAVIS

**TTP/HUS
AIHA**

GOODPASTURES
TRANSFUSION RXN (Rh⁺)

= → T4
GRAVES' DISEASE

IMMUNE DEPOSITION
CIRCULATING AG-AB COMPLEX
SYSTEMIC INVOLVEMENT
CLEAR AB/AG = CLEARS GOOD

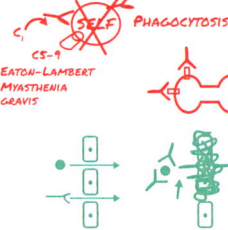

LUPUS ARTHUS
PSGN ABO

VASCULITIS, NEPHRITIS
ARTHRITIS

T-CELL MEDIATED = DELAYED HYPERSENSITIVITY
CTL (CD8) = CYTOKINES
$T_H 17$ = NEUTROPHILS
$T_H 1$ = MACROPHAGES CTL

PPD   * RA   CONTACT
CROHNS * MS   DERMATITIS
* CELIAC * GB

Transplant and Rejection

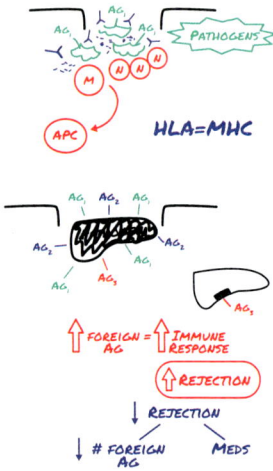

AG₁ AG₂ AG₃
PATHOGENS
M N N N
APC

HLA=MHC

AG₁ AG₂ AG₃
AG₂   AG₂
AG₁   AG₃
AG₃

↑ FOREIGN = ↑ IMMUNE
AG   RESPONSE

↑ REJECTION

↓ REJECTION

↓ # FOREIGN   MEDS
AG

GRAFTS

AUTOGRAFT DONOR = RECIPIENT
Ø REJECTION
TRANSFUSIONS, SKIN,
CABG

ISOGRAFT MONOZYGOTIC TWINS
DONOR ≈ RECIPIENT
SOMATIC MUTATIONS
REJECTION

ALLOGRAFT SAME SPECIES
(COMMON) BEST MATCH = ↓ REJECTION
↓ # FOREIGN AG

XENOGRAFT DIFFERENT SPECIES
PORCINE VALVE

A DONOR	B RECIPIENT	AB REJECT?
A	A	ACCEPTED
A	B ANTI-A	REJECTED
A	AB	ACCEPTED
AB	B ANTI-A	REJECTION

REJECTION

HYPERACUTE PREFORMED AB IGG
(MINS)   TYPE II ↳ THROMBOSIS

SCREEN = AB   PREVIOUSLY FAILED GRAFTS
TRANSFUSIONS

ACUTE   **T-CELL (IV)**
(DAYS)   ANTIGEN MISMATCH
THROMBOSIS, PARENCHYMAL
SCREEN = HLA MEDICATION, NONADHERENCE
AG   ↳ ANTI-REJECTION MEDS
             ↳ STEROIDS

CHRONIC
T-CELLS (IV) ⎫ FIBROSIS
B-CELL (II) ⎭

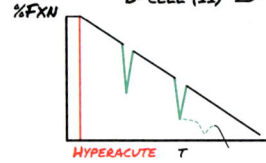

%FXN

HYPERACUTE   T

Immunology

Vaccines

"PASSIVE"
EXOGENOUS, SHORT-LIVED, RAPID ONSET

"NATURAL" HUMANS MAKE IT

N + P = IgG   PLACENTA | A + P = IVIg   "ARTIFICIAL" INJECT

N + A = (INFXN EXPOSURE) SURVIVE | A + A = VACCINE

"ACTIVE"
ENDOGENOUS, LONG-LIVED, SLOW ONSET

DIRTY WOUND

≥3 VACCINES ≤5 YRS AGO ✓

≥3 VACCINES TOXOID ≥5 YRS AGO

<3 VACCINES TOXOID ≥10 AGO IVIg

1ST EXPOSURE

IgM   MEMORY CELLS

0   10

SLOWER (7-10D)   1° AB RESPONSE   HIGHER / DOSE AG

WEAKER   ↓AFFINITY

TOXIN = DIE
TOXOID = IMMUNE

2ND EXPOSURE
IgG

0   4

FASTER (1-3)   2° AB RESPONSE   LOW DOSE AG

STRONGER   ↑AFFINITY

TOXIN = IMMUNE
TOXOID = IMMUNE / BOOSTER

IMMUNOGENIC
TOXOID
ANTIGENIC
TOXIN
DZ

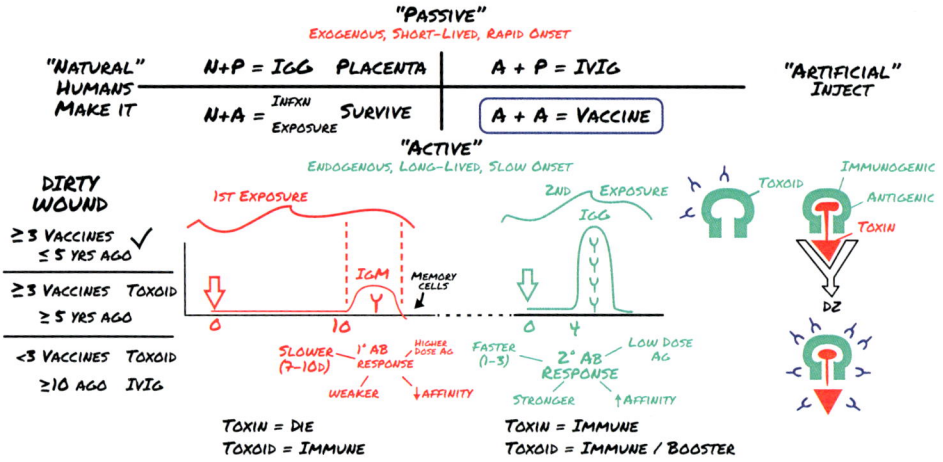

Mechanisms of Autoimmunity

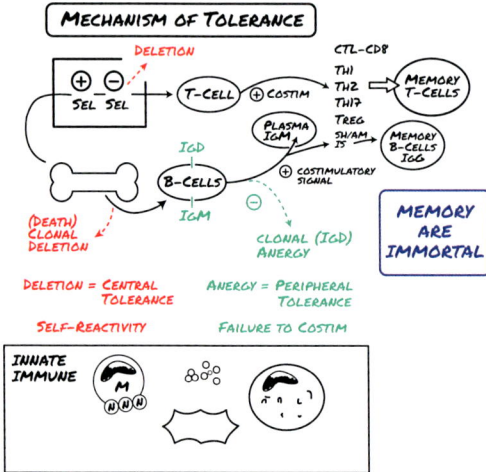

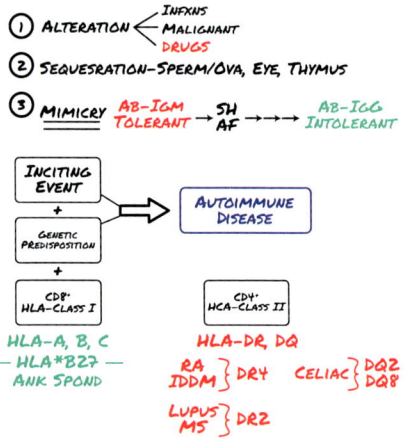

MECHANISM OF TOLERANCE

DELETION

⊕ ⊖
SEL SEL → T-CELL ⊕ COSTIM → MEMORY T-CELLS

CTL-CD8
TH1
TH2
TH17
TREG

IgD
PLASMA IgM   SW/AM IS → MEMORY B-CELLS IgG

B-CELLS   ⊕ COSTIMULATORY SIGNAL

IgM   ⊖

(DEATH) CLONAL DELETION

CLONAL (IgD) ANERGY

DELETION = CENTRAL TOLERANCE

ANERGY = PERIPHERAL TOLERANCE

SELF-REACTIVITY   FAILURE TO COSTIM

MEMORY ARE IMMORTAL

INNATE IMMUNE

① ALTERATION ← INFXNS / MALIGNANT / DRUGS

② SEQUESTRATION-SPERM/OVA, EYE, THYMUS

③ MIMICRY   AB-IgM TOLERANT → SW AF →→→ AB-IgG INTOLERANT

INCITING EVENT + GENETIC PREDISPOSITION +

CD8⁺ HLA-CLASS I

HLA-A, B, C
— HLA*B27 —
ANK SPOND

AUTOIMMUNE DISEASE

CD4⁺ HCA-CLASS II

HLA-DR, DQ

RA IDDM } DR4   CELIAC } DQ2 DQ8

LUPUS MS } DR2

Immunology

Immunosuppression

OnlineMedEd

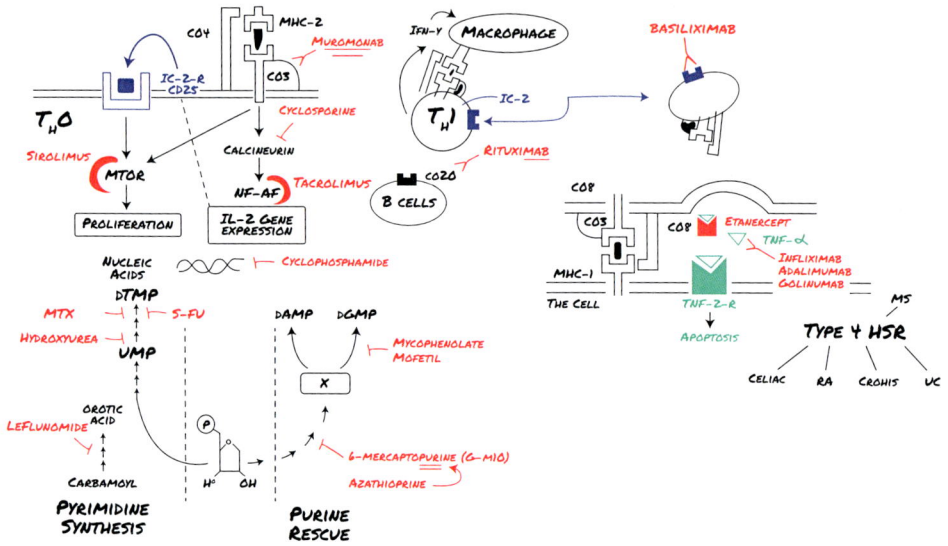

Immunology

Bacterial Structure and Intro

PLASMID

30S + 50S = 70S

CELL WALL

PEPTIDOGLYCAN

FLAGELLA = MOTILE

PILUS (PILI) FIMBRAE

PLASMA MEMBRANE

ENVELOPE TEICHOIC ACID

ENZYMES TOXINS

NUCLEOID DNA

LPS

CELL ENVELOPE

OUTER PLASMA MEMBRANE

PLASMA MEMBRANE

CELL ENVELOPE

ACID

GRAM ⊖   GRAM ⊕

ROD BACILLUS   CIRCLE COCCI

		ACID	
CRYSTAL VIOLET	PURPLE	–	PURPLE	
LIPID DETERGENT	PURPLE	–	COLORLESS	
SAFRANIN COUNTERSTAIN	PURPLE	–	PINK	
	⊕		⊖	

ADHESION — GRAM ⊖ PILI/ FIMBRAE / GRAM ⊕ TEICHOIC ACID / BIOFILMS

INVASION — HYALURONIDASE / COLLAGENASE ⎤ ECM / COAGULASE (STAPH AUREUS) / PHOSPHOLIPASE / PROTEASE ⎤ CELL

EVASION — CAPSULE ⟨ POLYSACCHARIDES / VACCINES / IGA PROTEASE / SPECIALIZATION

INTRACELLULAR — CATALASE / INHIBIT LYSOSOME FUSION / ESCAPE PHAGOSOME

EXTRACELLULAR — UREASE / OXIDASE / FERMENTATION SUGAR / SPORE

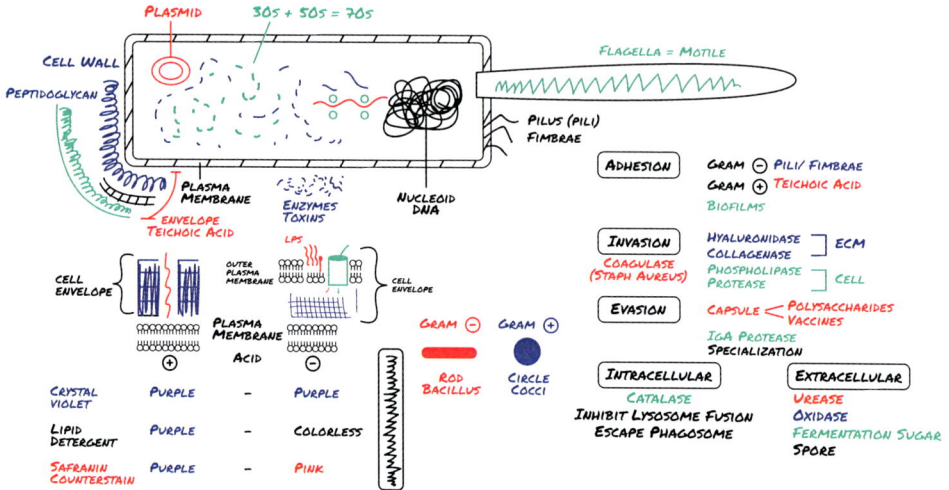

Bacterial Genetics

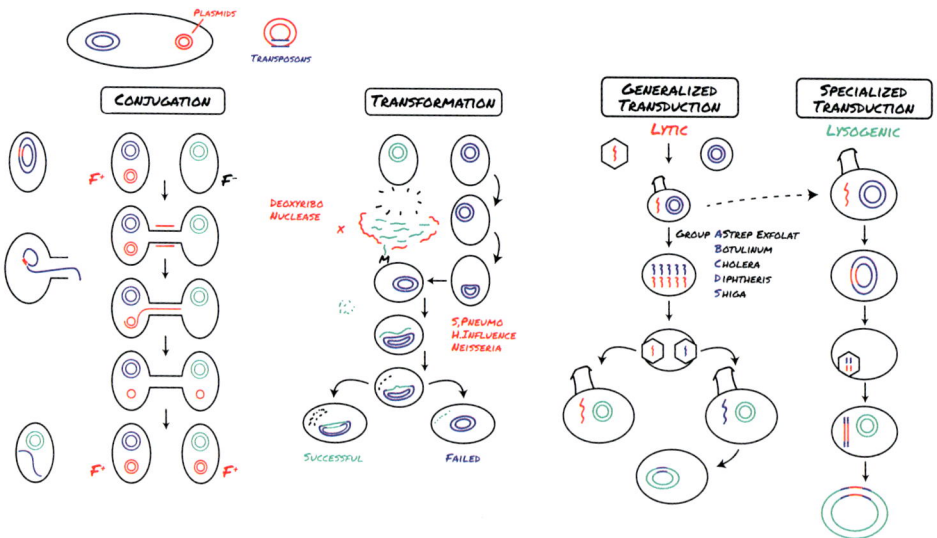

PLASMIDS

TRANSPOSONS

CONJUGATION

F⁺   F⁻

F⁺   F⁺

TRANSFORMATION

DEOXYRIBO NUCLEASE

X

M

S.PNEUMO H.INFLUENCE NEISSERIA

SUCCESSFUL   FAILED

GENERALIZED TRANSDUCTION

LYTIC

GROUP A STREP EXFOLAT BOTULINUM CHOLERA DIPHTHERIS SHIGA

SPECIALIZED TRANSDUCTION

LYSOGENIC

Bacterial Toxins

Output	Bacteria	Toxin	B Mechanism	A Target	Disease
Inhibit Protein Synthesis	C.Diphtheria	Diptheria	ADP-Ribosylation of EF-2	Oropharynx Hepatocytes	Diptheria, Gray Pseudomembrane Vaccine
	Pseudomonus	Exotoxin A			
	Shigella	Shiga	Removal of A from 60R rRNA	Enterocytes	Bloody Diarrhea HUS/TTP
	EHEC	Shiga-Like			
cAMP Inducers ↓ PKA ↓ Secretion	ETEC	HS-Toxin-cGMP HC-Toxin-cAMP	ADP-Ribsylation of Enterocytes GS → Activates AC → cAMP → PKA → Cl⁻	Watery diarrhea	
	B.Cereus	* HS-Toxin-cAMP HC-Toxin-cAMP		*Emesis Syndrome, S.Aureus Preformed Toxin	
	V. Chalerae	HC-Toxin-cAMP			
	Bordetella Pertussis	Pertussis	Gi Inactivating ADP-Ribosylation	Whooping Cough	Vaccine
Neurotoxins	Clostridium Tetoni	Tetanospasmin	Inhibit Synaptobrevin SNARE, Prevents Vehicle Fusion	Glycine/ GABA Ach	Tetanus – Lockjaw, Spastic Paralysis ↳ Rusty Wound Vaccine
	Clostridium Botulinum	Dotilism			Borulism – Flaccid Paralysis ↳ Floppy Baby – Honey – Home-Canned Goods
Kill Cells	Clostridium Perfringes	α – Toxin	Lecithinase	–	Myonecrosis = Gas Gangrene, Soil / Feces
	Strep Pyogenes	Streptolysin-O			
	Staph Aureus	Exfolatoxin			Scalded Skin Syndrome
Superantigens	Staph Aureus	TSST-1			Toxic Shack Syndrome, Nasal Packing Tampons
	Staph Pyogenes	Exotoxin A			

Laboratory Diagnosis

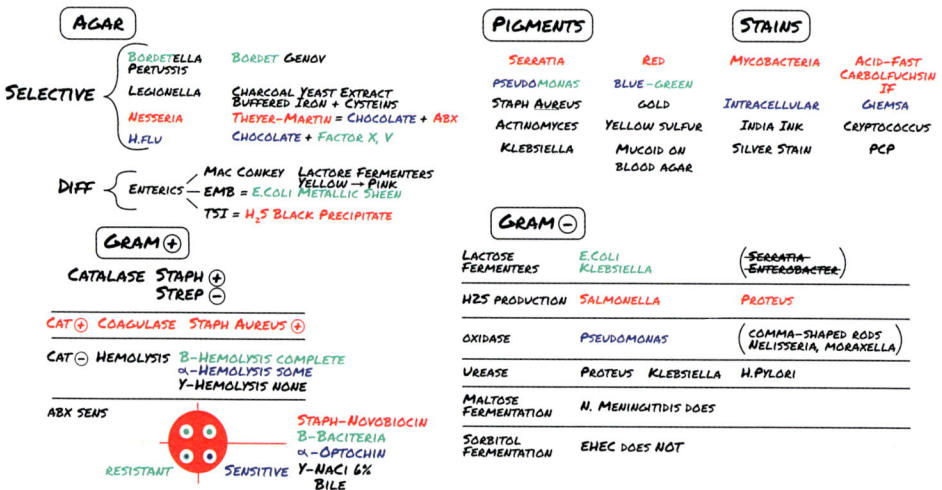

Agar

Selective
- Bordetella Pertussis → Bordet Genov
- Legionella → Charcoal Yeast Extract Buffered Iron + Cysteins
- Nesseria → Theyer-Martin = Chocolate + ABX
- H.Flu → Chocolate + Factor X, V

Diff { Enterics — Mac Conkey   Lactore Fermenters Yellow → Pink
— EMB = E.Coli Metallic Sheen
TSI = H_2S Black Precipitate

Gram ⊕

Catalase   Staph ⊕
Strep ⊖

Cat ⊕ Coagulase Staph Aureus ⊕

Cat ⊖ Hemolysis   B-Hemolysis complete
α-Hemolysis some
γ-Hemolysis none

ABX Sens

Staph–Novobiocin
B–Baciteria
α–Optochin
γ–NaCl 6%
Bile

Resistant   Sensitive

Pigments

Serratia	Red
Pseudomonas	Blue – Green
Staph Aureus	Gold
Actinomyces	Yellow Sulfur
Klebsiella	Mucoid on Blood Agar

Stains

Mycobacteria	Acid–Fast Carbolfuchsin
Intracellular	IF
India Ink	Giemsa
Silver Stain	Cryptococcus
	PCP

Gram ⊖

Lactose Fermenters	E.Coli Klebsiella	~~Serratia Enterobacter~~
H2S production	Salmonella	Proteus
Oxidase	Pseudomonas	Comma-Shaped Rods Nelisseria, Moraxella
Urease	Proteus Klebsiella	H.Pylori
Maltose Fermentation	N. Meningitidis does	
Sorbitol Fermentation	EHEC does NOT	

OME Bacterial Taxonomy

GRAM (+)

CIRCLE — SHAPE — rods — RODS — SPORE

SPORE FORMERS → O₂ → +O₂ → **BACILLUS**
- Anthracis
- B.Cereus (CIM)

−O₂ → **CLOSTRIDIUM**
- Perfringes (IM)
- Tetani
- Botulinum
- C.Diff

NON SPORE FORMERS → Branching → **BRANCHING**
- Actinocytes (−O₂)
- Nocardia

LEFT OVER
- Listeria
- Diphtheria

#6 — **COCCI**

COLONIES CATALASE

CLUSTERS CAT (+) — **STAPHS**

CHAINS CAT (−) — **STREPS**

COAGULASE
- (+) **STAPH AUREUS** — MRSA MSSA (t) [METHICILLIN]
- (−) **CONTAMINANT STAPHS** — Saprophyticus Epidermitis (t) [NOVOBICIN]

STREPS — HEMOLYSIS
- COMPLETE — **β-HEMOLYTIC STREPS** — Agalactae Pyogenes (t) [BACITRACIN]
- SOME — **α-HEMOLYTIC STREPS** — Viridans Pneumo (t) [OPTOCHIN]
- NO — **γ-HEMOLYTIC STREPS** — ENTEROCOCCUS [NaCl, BILE]

#14 **MYCOBACTERIA**
- Tuberculosis
- Leprosy
- MAC

GRAM (−)

SHAPE — rods — RODS — CIRCUMSTANCE

#7 **COCCI**
- N. Meningitis
- M. Gonorrhea
- Moraxella
- H. Influenae

#8 **DIARRHEA**
- Shigella
- Y.Enterocolitica
- Campylobacter
- EHEC
- ETEC
- V.Cholerae
- Salmonella Not Typhi
- Salmonella Typhi

#10 **ZOO**
- Yersinia Pestis (rats)
- F.Tularemis (rabbits)
- Brucella (dogs)
- Pasturella (cats)

#11 **SPIROCHETS**
- Syphilis Treponema Pallidum
- Lyme Borrelia Burgodorfei
- Leptospira

#12 **OBLIGATE INTRACELLULAR**
- Chlamydia Trachomatis
- Rickettsia – Rickettsia
  – Typhi
  – Prowazekii
- Bartonella
- Ealichia

#9 **EVERYONE ELSE**
- −O₂ → **ANAEROBES** (Bacteroides)
- +O₂ → **AEROBES** — Pseudomonas, Legionella

FACULTATIVE ANAEROBES

LACTOSE FERMENTERS
- YES → E.Coli Klebsiella
- NO → **PROTEUS**

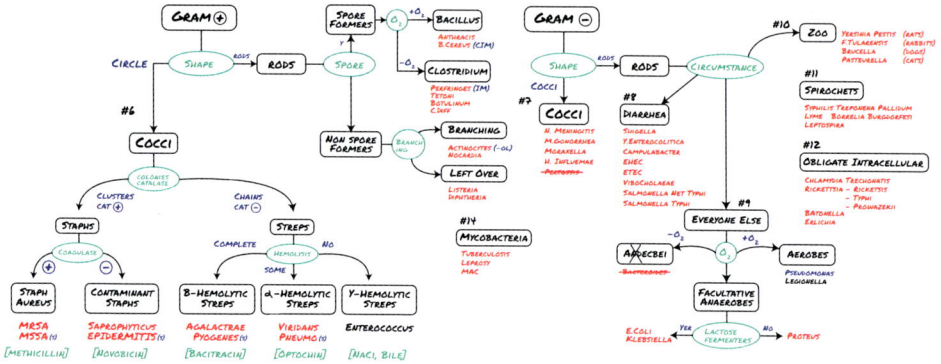

Gram-Positive Cocci

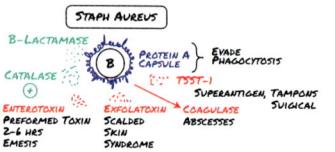

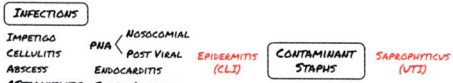

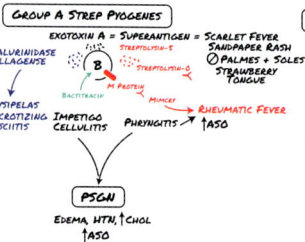

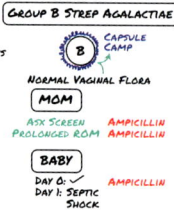

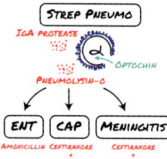

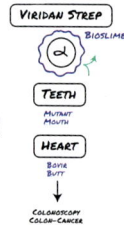

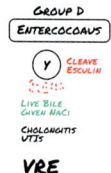

STAPH AUREUS

β-LACTAMASE

CATALASE (+)

PROTEIN A CAPSULE → EVADE PHAGOCYTOSIS

TSST-1 → SUPERANTIGEN, TAMPONS, SURGICAL

COAGULASE → ABSCESSES

ENTEROTOXIN — Preformed Toxin 2-6 Hrs Emesis

EXFOLATOXIN — Scalded Skin Syndrome

INFECTIONS
- IMPETIGO
- CELLULITIS
- ABSCESS
- OSTEOMYELITIS
- PNA — Nosocomial, Post Viral
- ENDOCARDITIS
- SEPTIC ARTHRITIS

EPIDERMITIS (CLI)

CONTAMINANT STAPHS

SAPROPHYTICUS (UTI)

GROUP A STREP PYOGENES

EXOTOXIN A = SUPERANTIGEN = SCARLET FEVER
- Sandpaper Rash
- ⊘ Palmes + Soles
- Strawberry Tongue

HYALURINIDASE COLLAGENSE

STREPTOLYSIN-S
STREPTOLYSIN-O

M Protein

MinCHF → RHEUMATIC FEVER ↑ASO

ERYSIPELAS NECROTIZING FASCIITIS — IMPETIGO CELLULITIS — Pharyngitis ↑ASO

PSGN — EDEMA, HTN, ↑CHOL ↑ASO

GROUP B STREP AGALACTIAE

CAPSULE CAMP

NORMAL VAGINAL FLORA

MOM — ASK SCREEN, PROLONGED ROM — AMPICILLIN AMPICILLIN

BABY — DAY 0: ✓ DAY 1: SEPTIC SHOCK — AMPICILLIN

STREP PNEUMO

IGA PROTEASE

OPTOCHIN

PNEUMOLYSIN-O
- **ENT** — Ampicillin Ceftriaxone + Acithro
- **CAP**
- **MENINGITIS** — Ceftriaxone + Vancomycin + Prednisone

VIRIDAN STREP

BIOSLIME

TEETH — Mutant Mouth

HEART — Bovie Butt — COLONOSCOPY COLON-CANCER

GROUP D ENTERCOCAUS

γ — CLEAVE ESCULIN

LIVE BILE GIVEN NaCl

CHOLONGITIS UTIS

VRE

NOTES

Gram-Negative Cocci

	Neisseria Meningitidis	Neisseria Gonorrhea (GC PCR)	Moraxella	Hemophilus
Micro	Gram ⊖ Diplococci Ferment Maltose	Gram ⊖ Diplococci –	Gram ⊖ Diplococci – Blood Agar	Gram ⊖ Coccobacillus – Chocolate Agar Factor X, V
CX	Theyer-Martin	Theyer-Martin	Respiratory	
Spread	Respiratory	STI		Respiratory
Virulence	Polysaccharide Capsule – Dx (Meningitis; Vaccine) Pili: Adhere (Vaccine) IgA Protease (Vaccine) Catastrophic Presentation Lipo-oligo-saccharide =	~~Capsule~~ Pili, Opa } Adherence (~~Vaccine~~) LPS	~~Capsule~~ LPS	Polysaccharide Capsule (Meningitis; Vaccine) Pili IgA Protease LPS
Dz:	Meningitis ↳ rapidly progressive 24 hrs ↳ Fever + Headache, Petechial Rash ↳ Adrenal Insufficiency, ↓BP + DIC	♀: Asx, Cerucitis PID Infertility, FHC ♂: Purulent Penile Discharge Reactive Arthritis Disseminated Gonorrhea Septic Arthritis	"Other other" Strep Pneumo #3 ENT: Sinusitis, Otitis Media CAP	"Other" Strep Pneumo #2 Epiglotitis: HIB Meningitis: HIB CAP-Copper Smoker
Tx:	Ceftriaxone PPX: Rifampin	Neonatal Blindness Ceftriaxone Azithro o, Doxy	Ceftriaxone Amoxicillin →	

Gram-Negative Rods - That Cause Serious Disease

	E.Coli	Klebsiella	Proteus	Pseudomonas	Legionella
Micro:	Lactose Fermenter – –	Lactose Fermenter Urease –	– Urease –	– – Oxidase	N/A BCYE Iron + Cystine
CX:	Metallic Green EMD	Mucoid Blood Agar	–	Blue - Green Colonies Grapes Smell Strict Aerobe	Loves H_2O
Virulence:	P-Pili ↳ UTI K, Capsule ↳ Neonatal Meningitis	Adherence Capsule	– –	Pyoverdin = green pig Pyocyocin = blue pig, superoxide dismutase Adhesions Capsule = Biofilms Exotoxin A (EF-2) Protease, Phosolipase, Elaste	Activates C3B-R ↓ Inhibits Lyososme Fusion
Dz:	UTI (MC) Neonatal Meningitis	UTI (2nd MC) ↳ Struvite Aspiration PNA ↳ Alcoholics ↳ Abscess ↳ Courant-Jelly Sputum	UTI ↳ Struvite Stones NH_4^+ Mg^{2+} P	Nosocomial PNA ↳ Hospitals, ventilators Burn Wounds ↳ "Tubbing" Penetration Sneaker ↳ Foot wounds, osteo Diabetic Foot Wounds ↳ Foot wounds, osteo UTI ↳ Indwelling Catheter ⇓ Cefepine, pip-tazo Carbapenen Monobactam Hot Tub ↳ Survive Cl Time Otitis Externa ↳ Swimmers Ear Corneal Ulcers ↳ Contacts ⇓ Ciprofloxacin gtts	Pontiac Fever ↳ Self-limiting febrile illness ↳ ∅ Dx Legionaires Dz ↳ PNA "(+)" GI + CNS Urinary Ag Macrolides

B:

SHIGELLA
LOW INOCULUM = FECAL-ORAL
  ↳ DAYCARE, MSM

M CELLS OF PEYER'S PATCHES
LYSES PHAGOSOME, CELL-TO-CELL

SHIGELLOSIS = BLOOD + PUS p̄ STRAINING
SHIGA TOXIN = DIAGNOSIS ←
  ↳ HUS ←

EHEC = STEC
LOW INOCULUM = FECAL-ORAL
  ↳ O157.H7 FROZEN BEEFS

COLONIC ENTEROCYTES

HEMORRHAGIC COLITIS
SHIGA TOXIN

EIEC] 3RD WORLD

Y. ENTEROCOLITICA
HIGH INOCULUM = PORK
  (PUPPY FECES)

ENTEROCYTES COLON, ILEUM
  ⊕ FEVER
BLOODY DIARRHEA
PSEUDOAPPENDICITIS

GROWS @ 4°C
COLDER MONTHS

CAMPYLOBACTER
HIGH INOCULUM = POULTRY
  (UNPASTEURIZED MILK)

ENTEROCYTES JEJUNUM, SUBMUCOSA
  ⊕ FEVER
BLOODY DIARRHEA
GUILLAIN-BARRE REACTIVE ARTHRITIS

GROWS @ 42°C BUT NOT @ 27°C
MICROAEROPHILIE (5% O₂)
COMMA-SHAPED,
RODS MOTILE, OXIDASE

SALMONELLA NOT TYPHI
HIGH INOCULUM = POULTRY, EGGS
  ↳ RAW CHICKEN, EGGS, PETS
       SNAKES, TURTLES
M CELLS OF PEYER'S PATCHES
LIVE WITHIN PHAGOSOME

SALMONELLOSIS   N/V/ WATERY DIARRHEA
       6-48 HRS p̄ INGESTION
       2-7 DAYS
       SELF LIMITING
OSTEOMYELITIS = SICKLE CELL DISEASE

SALMONELLA TYPHI
LOW INOCULUM = FECAL-ORAL
  ↳ IN HUMANS

M CELLS OF PEYER'S PATCHES

ENTERIC FEVER - TYPHOID
DAY 0: LIVER, SPLEEN, BM
       Ø DIARRHEA

DAY 14: GRADUAL ↑ FEVER
       FATIGUE, MALAISE, MYALGIAS
       ROX SPOTS ON TRUNK
       COLONIZE GALLBLADDER

DAY 2: COULD BE GI SXR

EIEC
HIGH INOCULUM = WATER
  ↳ TOXINS, TRAVELER'S

ADHERES TO ENTEROCYTES
TOXINS = DZ

SECRETORY DIARRHEA
       2-5 DAYS
       SELF-LIMITING

EPEC | 3RD WORLD
EAEL | INFANTS

VIBRIO CHOLERAE
HIGH INOCULUM = WATER
       ACID LABILE

ADHERES TO ENTEROCYTES
TOXINS = DZ

SECRETORY DIARRHEA
RICE-WATER STOCKS
       SELF-LIMITING

COMMA SHAPED RODS
OXIDASE ⊕, MOTILE

Gram-Negative Rods - Transmitted by Animals

YERSINIA PESTIS
THE BLACK DEATH

RATS CARRY FLEAS   ┐ RODENTS IN
FLEAS CARRY BACTERIA ┘ DESERT SW
(RAT BLOOD)   U.S.

CAPSULE PREVENTS
       LYSOSOME
       FUSION

- BUBONIC PLAGUE
70% FLEA BITES ANKLE, MACROPHAGES
MACROPHAGES → REGIONAL CN
BUBO → BACTEREMIC → DIC
       DEATH → GANGRONE

- PNEUMONIC PLAGUE (BIOTERRORISM)-
90% RAPIDLY PROGRESSIVE PNA
MEDIASTINAL CN

       GENTAMICIN

FRANCISELLA TULARENSIS
RABBIT PLAGUE

RABBIT CARRY TICKS
TICKS CARRY BACTERIA
RABBIT BLOOD BACTERIA

CAPSULE. PREVENTS
       LYSOSOME
       FUSION

- ULCEROGLANDULAR TULAREMIA
TICK BITES ANKLE, MACROPHAGES
MACROPHAGES → REGIONAL CN
"BUBO" → DEATH
ULCER @ BITE SITE

PNEUMONIC TULAREMIA
RABBIT HANDLING, PNA
WON'T IMPROVE
MEDIASTINAL CN

       GENTAMICIN

BRUCELLA
UNDULATING FEVER

ERYTHRITOL >> GLUCOSE
  ↳ BREAST - UNPASTEURIZED
              MILK
  ↳ UTERUS - DELIVERING
              CONSUMING PLACENTA
NO CAPSULE PREVENTS
       LYSOSOME
       FUSION

- BRUCELLOSIS
- SPLEEN, LIVER BM
THI = GRANULOMAS
TISSUE DESTRUCTION
HSM, ARTHRALGIAS, UNDULATING
FEVER
SERUM AB

DOXYCYCLINE +
RIFAMPIN

PASTEURELLA
ANIMAL BITES : CAT BITE FEVER

NORMAL FLORA CATS/DOGS
DOMESTICATED, PROVOKED = NONRABID
CAT WOUNDS = DEEP

CLEAN WOUND, DON'T SUTURE
AMOX-CLAV

BARTONELLA HENSELAE
CAT SCRATCH FEVER
CATS CARRY FLEAS
FLEAS CARRY BACTERIA

BABY HUMAN
CHRONIC LN p̄   ┐
KITTEN SCRATCH ├ SELF - LIMITING
"BABY" ABX   ┘

BACILLARY ANGIOMATOSIS
AIDS "ADULT"

Gram-Negative Rods - Spirochetes

Syphilis

TREPONEMA PALLIDUM = STI
1° PAINLESS ULCER + PAINFUL LN
~~CULTURE ANTIBODIES~~
DARKFIELD MICROSCOPY
IMMUNOFLUORESCENCE
   PENICILLIN G
   (DOXYCYCLINE)

2° MUCOCUTANEOUS COPPER COLORED
RASH DOES INVOLVE PALMS
+ SOLES
   NONTREPONEMAL — RPR 1:2
                   VRDL 1:1024
   FLUORESCENT TREPONEMA ANTIBODY
   ABSORPTION (FTA-ABS)
   PEN G / DOXYCYCLINE

LATENT ⊕ SEROLOGIES NO SXS
   DO REMEMBER = EARLY   PEN G
                 LATENT   DOXY
   DON'T REMEMBER = LATE   PEN G 9WK
                    LATENT 3 WKS

3° GUMMAS = GRANULOMATOUS
AORTA : AORTITIS, DISSECTION
BRAIN : "DEMENTIA"
        TABES DORSALIS
        ARGYL-ROBERTSON
CSF ANTIBODIES
PEN G x 1 WEEK

PREGNANT
CONGENITAL SYPHILLIS = BACTEREMIC
      (1° + 2° INFXN)
   Ø PCN ALLERGIC
   N/A = PCN
   ⊕ PCN ALLERGIC
1°, 2° : PCN DESENSITIZATION
   Ø : DEFER

J-H RXN
PCN → FEVER, CHILLS, LEUKEMIA
             RASH
   Ø PCN ALLERGIC

Lyme, CT

BORRELIA BURGDORFERI = TICK BORNE
IXODER TICK IS VECTOR
WHITE FOOTED MOUSE, WHITE-TAILED DEER
EXPOSURE TO TICKS
~~VISUALIZED/ REMOVED TICK~~   N.E.
                                 U.S
PHASE I   HIKING W/ 1 MONTH
EARLY   RASH = TARGETS : D
LYME   FEVER, ARTHRALGIAS, MALAISE ETC.
          DOXYCYCLINE

PHASE II   PHASE FOR 1 MONTH
INVASIVE   INVASION + BACTEREMIA
LYME
   NERVES   HEART   CNS
(BELL'S PALSY) (BLOCKS) (MENINGITIS)
          SEROLOGY ⊕
          IV CEFTRIAXONE

PHASE III LYME ARTHRITIS
LATE   NEVER BEEN TREATED
LYME   IMPRESSIVE OFFUSIONS
          SEROLOGY ⊕
          IV CEFTRIAXONE
CHRONIC
LYME   ARTHRITIS Ƥ ABX
         IS SOMETHING ELSE

Leptospirosis

LIVER IN ANIMALS
INFECTS HUMANS
(WATER SKIING)

1 PHASE : LEPTOSPREMIC
2 PHASE : IMMUNE
   * WEIL'S SYNDROME
   LIVER
   JAUNDICE
   ↑LFTS

   FHF 10%

Gram-Negative Rods - Intracellular Obligate Parasites

Chlamydia Trachomatis A-L

HUMAN VECTOR
UBIQUITOUS WORLDWIDE
ENERGY PARASITES
W/I PHAGOSOME, NON-CILIATED EPITHELIUM

- TRACHOMA = A, B, C AFRICAN BLINDNESS CHILDREN
   ACUTE FOLLICULITIS
   RECURRENT FOLLICULITIS = SCARRING
   ABX + HAND / FACE HYGENE
   KIDS ARE COLONIZED, SPREAD

- UROGENITAL = U.S. = D-K
   ♀ : ASX, CERVICITIS, PID, INFERTILITY
       MOST COMMON BACTERIAL STI ~~WET MOUNT~~
   ♂ : THICK WHITE PURULENT D/C ~~EX~~
       AZITHROMYCIN OR DOXY ← GC
                               PCR
                               URINE

- LGV = L1, L2, L3
   - PAINLESS ULCER THEN PAINFUL NODE
   - GRANUMBMAS ... OBSTRUCTION OF SYMPHATICS
                    GENITAL ELEPHANTIASIS
   - NODER   - ULCER ABOVE NODE
     RUPTURE SINUS DRAINING TRACK

Rickettsia

ARTHOPOD VECTOR

ENERGY PARASITES
CYTOPLASM, ENDOTHELIAL CELLS

- ROCKY MOUNTAIN SPOTTED FEVER = RICKETTSII
- TICK BORNE DZ ENDEMIC EXPOSURE APPALACHIAN
- EXPOSURE TO TICKS, ~~SEE A LICH~~
- UNAWARE → FEVER + → RASH WRISTS/ ANKLES → DOXYCYCLINE
  OF TICK   HEADACHE   SPREADS EVERYWHERE   AGE AGNOSTIC
  (7 DAYS)   (2DAYS)   INCLUDING PALMS/ SOLES

          "MENINGITIS"   "DRUG RXN"
          CEFTRIAXONE
             +
          VANCOMYCIN
- ENDOTHELIAL CELLS → SMALL VESSLE VASCULITIS

EPIDEMIC TYPHUS PROWAZEKII   EPIDEMIC TYPHUS TYPHI
HUMAN LOUSE   RATS, RAT FLEAS

UNAWARE →   FEVER + →   PINK MAWLER, STOUT OP TRUNK
TRANSMISSION   HEADACHE   DESCENDING LIMBS
(7 DAYS)   (2 DAYS)

[graph] =ACUTE/ SEVERE   [graph] =SUBACUTE
                                    NON SEVERE

LARGE VESSELS
GANGRENE, THROMBOSIS

118

© 2020 OnlineMedEd

Gram-Postive Rods

Bacillus (+)

SPORES:
- **Anthracis**
- **Cereus** — Ae
- **Clostridia** — AN
- **Perferingens**
- **Tetani**
- **Botulinum**
- **Difficile**

Capsule → NO | Immotile → Motile
Immotile → Motile

Anthrax
Bacillus Anthracis polypeptide Capsule
Exotoxins → Protective / Edema / Lethal
Ciprofloxacin or Doxycycline

Cutaneous 95% Papule → Pustule + Painful Painless LN
Black
Pulmonary 5% PNA + Mediastinal Hemorrhagic Lymphadenitis

B. Cereus
B.Cereus — GI Reheated Rice/ Buffet cines
- Heat Stable = Emesis
- Heat Labile = Diarrhea

C. Diff Colitis
C. Diff = Normal Flora
- Toxin A = Enterotoxin → Water Diarrhea
- Toxin B = Cytotoxin → Bloody Diarrhea

C. Diff Colitis (Overgrowth, ABX Clinda)
- Pseudomembrane Colitis
- Megacolon, Paralytic Ileus
- Profuse watery Diarrhea
Toxin, PCR

Gas Gangrene
- C.Perferingens → Enterotoxin
- α Toxin = Lecithinase Destroys Membranes Host Cells

Contaminated wounds by soil or feces

Ferment sugars to CO_2

Tetanus
C. Tetani. Tetanospasm inhibits inhibitory neuron (GABA/Gly)
Wound Rusty Soil
(DTap)
Trismus (Lock Jaw)
Risus Sardonicus
Sapstic Paralysis

Cellulitis + Crepitus/ "Air"
CLINDAMYCIN = ↓ Toxin (Translation-J)

Synaptobrevin Protease Vesicle Can't Fuse

Botulism
C. Botulinum (ACH)
Adult Form: Home canned food, Poorle Reheat, Preformed heat labile toxin (ACH)
Flappy Baby: Spores in honey ingested → Toxin
Flaccid Paralysis

C. Diff TX
1. Mild-Mod, 1st PO VANC IV VANC
2. Mild-Mod, 2nd PO VANC IV VANC
3. Mild-Mod, 3rd PO VANC... Fidaxomicin
4. Refractory Fecal Transplant
5. Severe PO VANC + IV MTZ

NO SPORES:
- **Listeria** — Ae
- **Diphtheria**
- **Nocardia**
- **Actinomyces** — AN

No Capsule | Motile
Flagella Protein Rocket
Immotile

Branching	+ Acid Fast	Soil Cavitary Lung Lesions
Branching	+ ∅	Normal Oral Flora / Sulfur Draining Tracts

Facultative Intracellular Grow @ 0°C Grow @ 4°C
Pseudomembrane (DTap)
Moms Deli Meat/ Cheese Inutero = Progenic, Lost of Preg Neonatal Meningitis

---

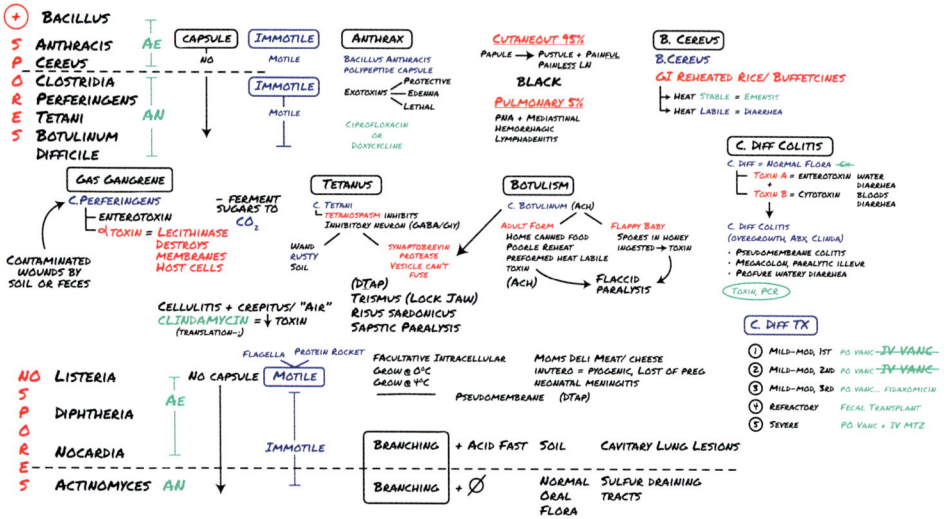

Mycobacterium

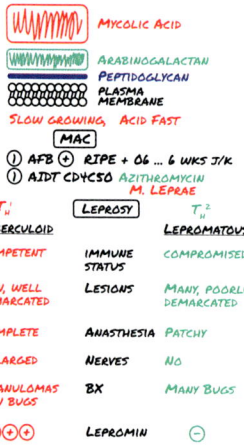

Mycobacteria
- Mycolic Acid
- Arabinogalactan Peptidoglycan
- Plasma Membrane
Slow Growing, Acid Fast

MAC
1. AFB ⊕ RIPE + O6 ... 6 wks J/k
2. AIDT CD4<50 Azithromycin

M. Leprae

Leprosy

T_H^1 Tuberculoid		T_H^2 Lepromatous
Competent	Immune Status	Compromised
Few, well demarcated	Lesions	Many, poorly demarcated
Complete	Anasthesia	Patchy
Enlarged	Nerves	No
Granulomas Few Bugs	BX	Many Bugs
⊕⊕⊕	Lepromin	⊖

Tuberculosis — M. Tuberculosis

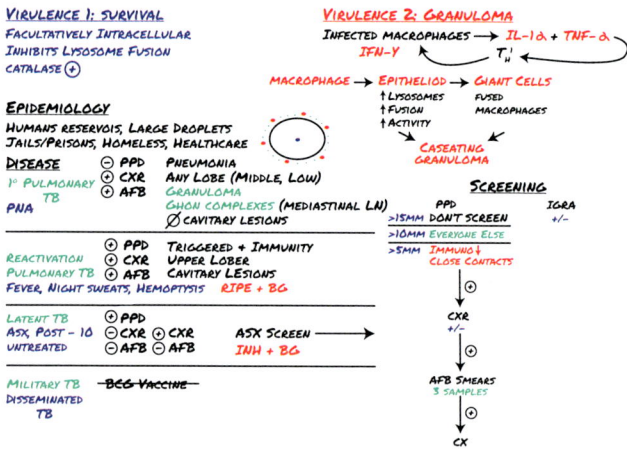

Virulence 1: Survival
Facultatively Intracellular
Inhibits Lysosome Fusion
Catalase ⊕

Epidemiology
Humans reservoir, Large droplets
Jails/Prisons, Homeless, Healthcare

Disease
1° Pulmonary TB / PNA
- ⊖ PPD: Pneumonia
- ⊕ CXR: Any Lobe (Middle, Low)
- ⊕ AFB: Granuloma / Ghon Complexes (Mediastinal LN) / ∅ Cavitary Lesions

Reactivation Pulmonary TB
Fever, Night Sweats, Hemoptysis
- ⊕ PPD: Triggered + Immunity
- ⊕ CXR: Upper Lober
- ⊕ AFB: Cavitary Lesions
RIPE + B6

Latent TB ASX, Post - 10 Untreated
- ⊕ PPD
- ⊖ CXR ⊖ CXR
- ⊖ AFB ⊖ AFB
ASX Screen → INH + B6

Military TB Disseminated TB — BCG Vaccine

Virulence 2: Granuloma
Infected Macrophages → IL-1α + TNF-α
IFN-γ ⇄ T_H^1
Macrophage → Epitheliod → Giant Cells
↑Lysosomes ↑Fusion ↑Activity / Fused Macrophages
Caseating Granuloma

Screening
PPD
- >15mm Don't Screen
- >10mm Everyone Else
- >5mm Immuno↓ Close Contacts
IGRA +/-

CXR +/-
AFB Smears 3 Samples ⊕
CX

120 © 2020 OnlineMedEd

Introduction to Antibacterials

β-Lactam Cell Wall Inhibitors

NOTES

Cell Wall Inhibitors Not β-Lactams

OnlineMedEd

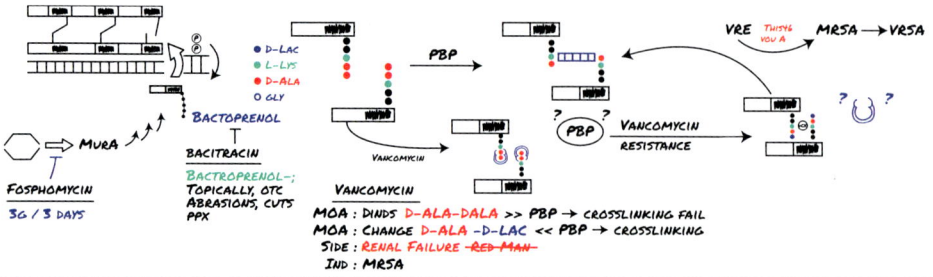

Translation Inhibitors

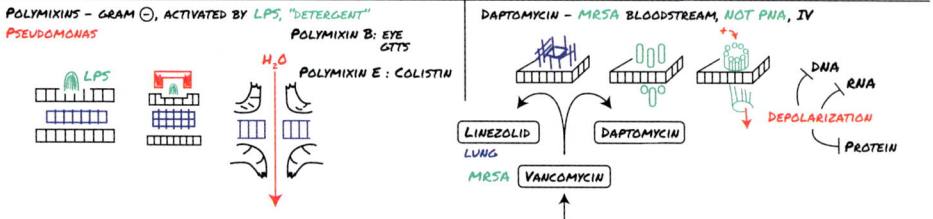

DNA and RNA Inhibitors

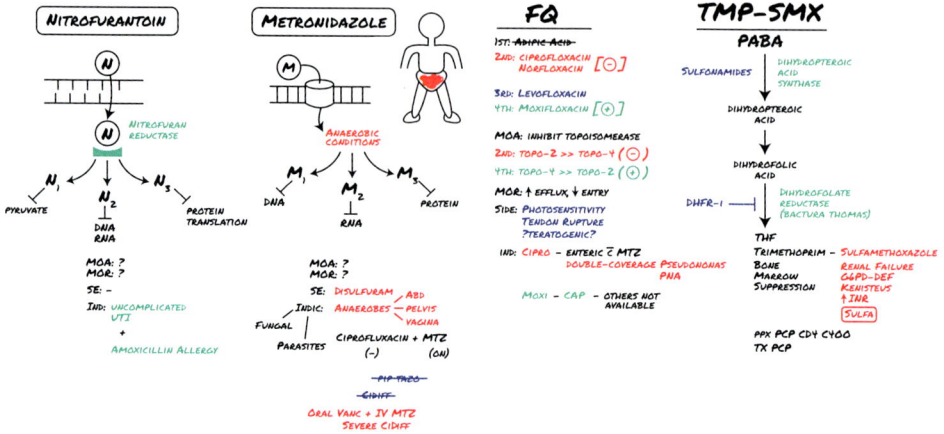

Antimycobacterial

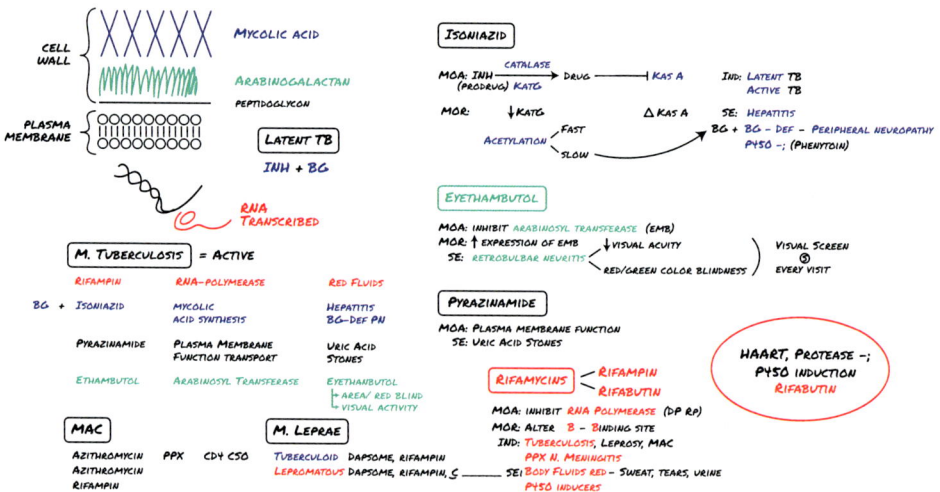

Introduction to Viruses

VIRION
VIRUS = GENOME — DNA
+ RNA } NUCLEOCAPSID
CAPSID
+ ENVELOPE

TEMPLATE
5'
3' C T A T
5' G A U A 3'
5' G A T A
3'
CODING

DNA VIRUSES
GCAT
NUCLEUS
HOST POLYMERASES
DSDNA

5' MG 3'
AAA

5'— VIRUS —3' SS(+)RNA
5'— ƧUЯIV —3' SS(−)RNA

RNA VIRUSES
GCAU
CYTOPLASM
SSRNA
VIRAL POLYMERASES

NAKED
ICOSAHEDRAL

ENVELOPED
ICOSAHEDRAL

HELICAL

CYTOPLASM
TF, ENZYMES

GLYCOPROTEINS

HOST CELL
PLASMA
MEMBRANE

DNA POLYMERASE
(REPLICATION)

HUMAN
MAKER
(POLYMERASE)

RNA POLYMERASE
(TRANSCRIPTION)

READS DNA
(DEPENDENT)

DNA

DDDP

RNA

DDRP

RNA

REVERSE
TRANSCRIPTURE

RDDP

RDRP

VIRAL

ALL RNA
VIRUSES

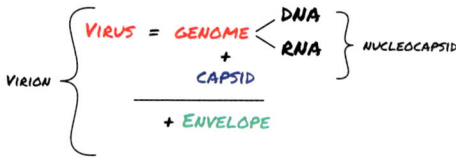

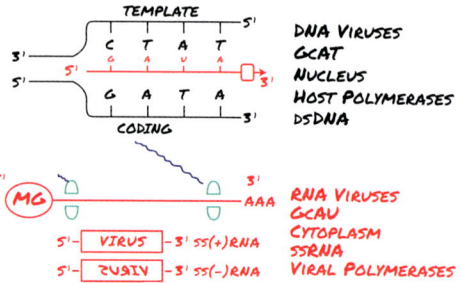

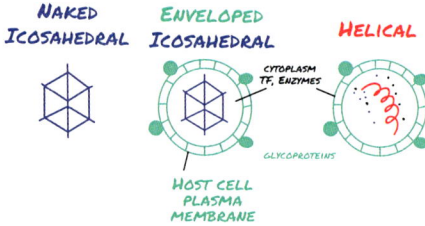

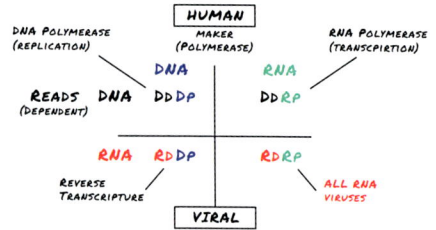

Life Cycle of Viruses

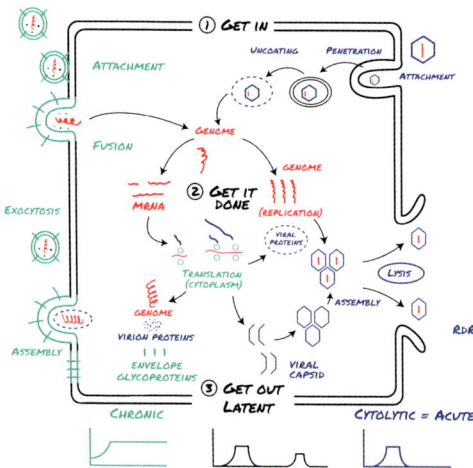

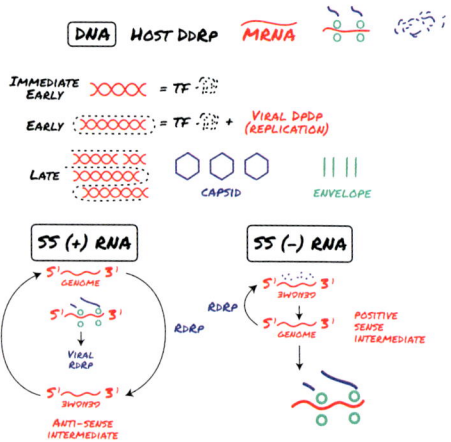

① GET IN

ATTACHMENT

UNCOATING   PENETRATION

ATTACHMENT

FUSION

GENOME

GENOME

EXOCYTOSIS

MRNA

② GET IT
DONE (REPLICATION)

VIRAL
PROTEINS

LYSIS

TRANSLATION
(CYTOPLASM)

ASSEMBLY

GENOME

VIRION PROTEINS

ASSEMBLY

ENVELOPE
GLYCOPROTEINS

VIRAL
CAPSID

RDRP

③ GET OUT
LATENT

CHRONIC

CYTOLYTIC = ACUTE

DNA HOST DDRP MRNA

IMMEDIATE
EARLY   = TF

EARLY   = TF + VIRAL DPDP
(REPLICATION)

LATE

CAPSID   ENVELOPE

SS (+) RNA

5' 3'
GENOME

5' 3'

VIRAL
RDRP

5' 3'
GENOME

ANTI-SENSE
INTERMEDIATE

RDRP

RDRP

SS (−) RNA

5' 3'
GENOME

5' 3'
GENOME

POSITIVE
SENSE
INTERMEDIATE

DNA Viruses

NAKED
DSDNA
NUCLEUS
ICOSAHEDRAL

DNA
VIRUSES

~~HEPATITIS~~
HERPES
HAVE ENVELOPE

PARVOVIRUS
B19

INFXN → FEVER → ASX

SSDNA
TINY

ERYTHROID   ERYTHEMA
PRECARIOUS   INFECTIOSUM

SCD = APLASTIC ANEMIA

HPV

PERSISTENT INFXN = LYSIS TOP LAYER

GRAVES →
GRANULOSUM
SPINOSUM
BASAL

MUCOSAL HPV
(SCC)

THROAT   ANUS   CERVIX

CANCER
16, 18
PAP SMEARS
9-VALENT = 16, 18, 6, 11
VACCINES + 5 OTHERS

CUTANEOUS HPV
(SCC)

GENITAL   SKIN

WARTS
6, 11   1, 2, 4
IMIQUIMOD
CIDOFOVIR

ADENOVIRUS

ACUTE INFXN

FECCI - ORAL
OROPHARYNX
AEROSOLS

PINK EYES   DIARRHEA

INFECTION → NUCLEUS → IE: TF FOR E
                      E: VIRAL DDDP (REPLICATION)
LATS   LATENCY   THYMIDINE KINASE
       RNA   C: CAPSID ENVELOPE

HHU-1, 2   HSV   VESICLES ON AN ERYTHEMATOUS
                 BASE, PAINFUL PRODROME
                 ACUTE = MUCO
                              CUTANEOUS = LOCAL
                 LATENT = NEURONS

FEVER BLISTERS/ COLD SORES HSV-1
HSV ENCEPHALITIS HSV-1
GENITAL VICERS HSV1 = HSV-2
ACYCLOVIR

HHU-3   VZV   SAA
              ACUTE = CUTANEOUS = DISSEMINATED
              LATENT = NEURONS
              ACYCLOVIR

CHICKENPOX   DISSEMINATED
VACCINE   CROPS
              SEPARATED
SHINGLES   DERMATOMAL
              CRAMPED

HHU-4   EBV   INFECTIOUS MONONUCLEOSIS = KISSING DISEASE
        LIVER FEVER, SORE THROAT, EXUDATES, LN, HSM, RASH
               BLOOD SMEAR = BOUNCY CELLS HETEROPHILE AB ⊕
               LATENT = B CELLS = BURKITTS, HODGKINS

HHU-5   CMV   HETEROPHILE AB ⊖ MONO
        BRAIN CONGENITAL CMV = VISION/HEARING, MR, INTRACEREBAL
        EYE   AIDS = DISSEMINATE   INCLUSIONS
MILITARY   LATENT - MONOCYTES
ORAL
VACCINE

HHV6-7   ROSEOLA   HHV8   KAPOSI SARCOMA

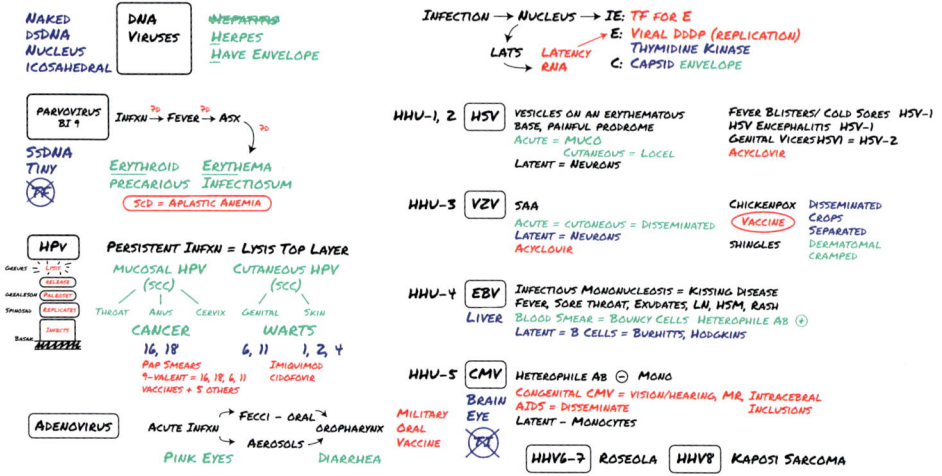

ss(+)RNA Viruses

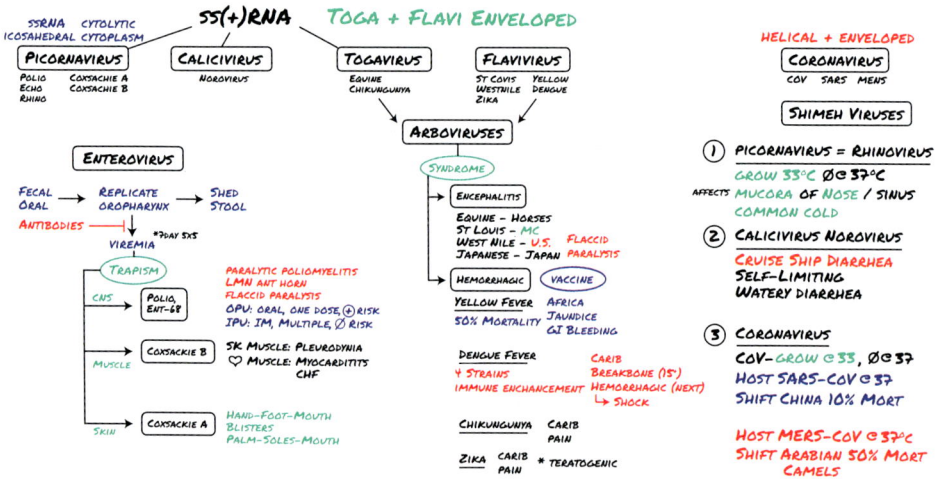

SSRNA   CYTOLYTIC
ICOSAHEDRAL CYTOPLASM

ss(+)RNA   TOGA + FLAVI ENVELOPED

PICORNAVIRUS   CALICIVIRUS   TOGAVIRUS   FLAVIVIRUS

POLIO COXSACHIE A   NOROVIRUS   EQUINE   ST COVIS   YELLOW
ECHO   COXSACHIE B   CHIKUNGUNYA   WESTNILE   DENGUE
RHINO   ZIKA

ARBOVIRUSES

SYNDROME

ENTEROVIRUS

FECAL → REPLICATE → SHED
ORAL   OROPHARYNX   STOOL
ANTIBODIES   *7DAY SXS
            VIREMIA

TRAPISM

CNS   POLIO,
       ENT-68

MUSCLE   COXSACKIE B

SKIN   COXSACKIE A

PARALYTIC POLIOMYELITIS
LMN ANT HORN
FLACCID PARALYSIS
OPU: ORAL, ONE DOSE, ⊕ RISK
IPU: IM, MULTIPLE, ∅ RISK

SK MUSCLE: PLEURODYNIA
♡ MUSCLE: MYOCARDITITS
CHF

HAND-FOOT-MOUTH
BLISTERS
PALM-SOLES-MOUTH

ENCEPHALITIS
EQUINE - HORSES
ST LOUIS - MC
WEST NILE - U.S.   FLACCID
JAPANESE - JAPAN   PARALYSIS

HEMORRHAGIC   VACCINE
YELLOW FEVER   AFRICA
50% MORTALITY JAUNDICE
               GI BLEEDING

DENGUE FEVER   CARIB
4 STRAINS   BREAKBONE (1S)
IMMUNE ENHANCEMENT   HEMORRHAGIC (NEXT)
                         → SHOCK

CHIKUNGUNYA   CARIB
              PAIN

ZIKA   CARIB   * TERATOGENIC
       PAIN

HELICAL + ENVELOPED

CORONAVIRUS
COV   SARS   MENS

SHIMEH VIRUSES

① PICORNAVIRUS = RHINOVIRUS
   GROW 33°C ∅ⓒ 37°C
AFFECTS MUCOA OF NOSE / SINUS
   COMMON COLD

② CALICIVIRUS NOROVIRUS
   CRUISE SHIP DIARRHEA
   SELF-LIMITING
   WATERY DIARRHEA

③ CORONAVIRUS
   COV- GROW ⓒ 33, ∅ⓒ 37
   HOST SARS-COV ⓒ 37
   SHIFT CHINA 10% MORT

   HOST MERS-COV ⓒ 37°C
   SHIFT ARABIAN 50% MORT
   CAMELS

OnlineMedEd

SS(-)RNA

PARAMYXOVIRUS	RHABDOVIRUS	~~FITO~~	ORTHOMYXOVIRUS	~~BUNYA~~	~~ARONA~~
RSV MEASLES	RABIES	~~EBOLA~~	FLU	~~HARTA~~	~~LARRA FEVER~~
PARAINF MUMPS		~~MABURO~~			

RESPIRATORY DROPLETS

ATTACH   RELEASE
HEMAGGLUTININ   NEURAMINIDASE
       OSELTAMIVIR

H1:N1
ANNUAL VACCINE
IM KILLED →
~~EGGS~~
72 HRS

PARAMYXO PULM

GROUP (PARAINF)
SEAL-LIKE BARKING
COUGH
SELF-LIMITING
4-7 YRS

BRONCHIOLITIS (RSV)
"ASTHMA, CLYO, ⊕ FEVER"

WHEEZING

~~RIBAVIRUS~~

PARAMYXO RASH

MEASLES : RESP EPITH
COUGH   VIREMIA = FEVER
CORYZA
CONJUNCTIVITY   PRODROME
PHOTOPHOBIA
       SPORTS / CAPLITE
MMRU

RASH EARS → BODY
SSPE   ??
MUMPS : ORCHITIS
       PARODITIS
       INFERTILITY

ORTHAMYXOVIRUS

      ANTIGENIC DRIFT
SEGMENTED ⟨
      ANTIGENIC SHIFT

REPLICATE   NUCLEUS
       OR
       CYTOPLASM

FLU SEASON : FALL TO SPRING
FLU SXS : MYALGIAS, FEVER / CHILLS, NIV, HIA

RHABDOVIRUS

SK MUSCLE   ① INCUBATION PHASE
REPLICATING   30 - 60 DAYS

ASCENDING   ② PRODOME
NEURON   PAIN @ BTE SITE
         7-14D

GLANDS   ③ NEUOLOGIC
URINE   PHASE
        AMS, FEAR OF WATER, CUMA

DX: ANIMAL → NEGRI
    RNA URINE   TOO LATE
    ECISA   TOO LATE

TX: ANTIBODY
    VACCINE

HIV and AIDS

P24
GENOME SS(+)RNA
INTEGRASE
REVERSE TRANSCRIPTASE
PROTEASE
GP120
GP41

CD4
CCR5*
CXCR*

RDDP
EXO
DDDP

VIRAL
LOAD

HIV-AB

P24

10	20	30	40	50	60

ECLIPSE   ACUTE   3RD GEN   2ND GEN   1ST GEN

HIV PCR   P24 + HIV-AB → HIV-1
               HIV-2

ENV	GP120	ATTACHMENT
	GP41	FUSION
POL	PRO	PROTEASE
	POL	RT
	INT	INTEGRASE
GAG	P24	IDENTIFICATION

PRO POL INT
GP41 GP120   P24
PROTEASE   mRNA   mRNA   GENOME
       DDRP   INTEGRASE
DDRP

ASSESS: CD4   VIRAL   GENOTYPING
       COUNT   LOAD   (RESISTANCE)
       (NOW)   (GOING)

CD4	BUG	PPX	HAART
C200	PCP	TMP-SMX	"2+1"
<100	TOXO	TMP-SMX	
<50	MAC	AZITHROMYCIN	

ROUTES

BLOOD	IVDA*
	TATTOO
	NEEDLESTICK
	BLOOD TRANSFUSION
SEX	VAGINAL
	ANAL
PERI	VERTICAL TRANSMISSION
NATAL	INTRAUTERINE
	BREAST MILK

SXS

① ACUTE RETROVIRAL SYNDROME
    FEVER, SORE THROAT, LN

② LATENT
    ASX
    INFECTIOUS

③ AIDS
    CD4 < 200
    OPPORTUNISTIC
    INFXNS

IFN-γ
IL-17
B-CELL   CD4G-L   NEUTROPHILS
      CDLB
        CD4
IL 3, 4, 5
MAST CELLS   IL-2 → CD8 CYTO
EOSINOPHILS
IGE

Hepatitis Viruses

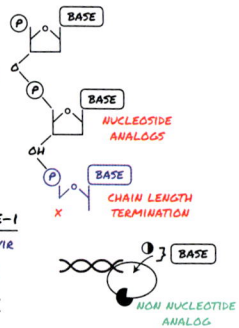

HEP A	HEP B	HEP C	HEP D	HEP E
FECAL-ORAL	SEX VERTICAL BLOOD	BLOOD = NEEDLES	SEX VERTICAL BLOOD	FECAL - ORAL
NAKED	ENVELOPED ACUTE: ↑LFT	ENVELOPED	"ENVELOPED" (HEP B)	NAKED
ACUTE INFXN MODERATE HEPATITIS + DIARRHEA	BOTH JAUNDICE, CLEAR / CHRONICS Ø SXS, NOT CLEAR	CHRONIC CIRRHOSIS HCC	CO-INFECTION = WORSE B SUPER = FHF INFECTION	ACUTE INFXN MILD X̄ PREGNANT WOMAN
PICORNAVIRUS SS(+)RNA ICOSAHEDRAL	HEPADNAVIRUS INCAPABLE DSDNA ICOSAHEDRAL	FLAVIVIRUS SS(+)RNA ICOSAHEDRAL	SS(+)RNA VIRUS ICOSAHEDRAL	CALICIVIRUS SS(+)RNA ICOSAHEDRAL
VACCINE ⊕ (KILLED HEP A)	VACCINE ⊕ (HEPBS AG)	CORE (DAA)	HepB CAG SAG	NO VACCINE
US: CONTAMINATED FOOD	ASIA: VERTICAL US: SEX	US: IVDA	EAG → PLASMA	3RD WORLD

AG / AG AG AG = VACCINE

ANTI-HBs = IMMUNE   Ø ANTI-HBs = Ø IMMUNE

EXPOSURE | VACCINE   NO | ⊕   EARLY / UNDECIDED | LATE/ CHRONIC
ANTI-HBc | _____   AG | AG   ANTI-HBc IgM ⊕ | ANTI-HBc IgM ⊕
                                          IgG, -   IgG, ⊕

Antivirals

HERPESVIRUS

(VAL) ACYCLOVIR   HSV, VZV, EBV, "G", THYMIDINE KINASE , BONE MARROW ↓
(VAL) GANCICLOVIR   CMV   , "G", TK, PHOSPHOTRANSFERASE , BONE MARROW ↓
FOSCARNET   ALL, NONNUCLEOTIDE, IV NEPHROTOXICITY

P — BASE
P — BASE   NUCLEOSIDE ANALOGS
OH
X — BASE   CHAIN LENGTH TERMINATION
BASE   NON NUCLEOTIDE ANALOG

HIV   "2 + 1"
NRT-1   ANY OTHER CLASS   -NAVIR (PRO)

NRT-1	NNRT-1	PROTEASE-1	ENTRY-1	-TEGRA- INTEGRASE-1
TENOFAVIR(R) EMTRICITABINE	EFAVIRENZ(T)	ATAZANAVIR/r(S) DARUNAVIR/r RITONAVIR	MARAVISOL (CCR5) GP120 ENFURVITIDE (GP41)	RAL-TEGRA-VIR
LAMIVUDINE ZIDOVUDINE (ART=PREGNANCY)	RELPIVIRINE NEVIRAPINE			
ABACAVIR = HSR = 5% FATAL DIDANOSINE = 30% PANCREATITIS				

HEP B   INTERFERON X RIBAVIRIN "G"

REVERSE TRANSCRIPTASE
TENOFAVIR   2 MEDS
ADEFOVIR
LAMIVUDINE "C"
ENTACAVIR "G"

HEP C   INTERFERON X RIBAVIRIN   RDRP = NS5B

DIRECT ACTING ANTAGONISTS   2 MECHANISMS

-UVIR   SOFOSUVIR - NS5B - NUCLEOTIDE ANALOG -1
         DASABUVIR - NS5B - NONNUCLEOTIDE ANALOG -1

-PREVIR _____ - NS³4A - PROTEASE -1

-ASVIR   LEDIPASVIR - NS5A-1 - ASSEMBLY

EUKARYOTIC — NUCLEUS, MITOCHONDRIA, 80D RIBOSOME

PLASMA MEMBRANE – ERGOSTEROL

CELL WALL – CHITIN, B-GLUCAN

KAT PREP | LACTOL PHENOL BLUE | SABOURAUD AGOR

YEASTS | MOLDS

BLASTO COMIDIA | COMIDA | ARTHRO COMIDO (SPORE)

PSEUDOBYPHAE | SEPTATE 45° | NON SEPTATE 90°

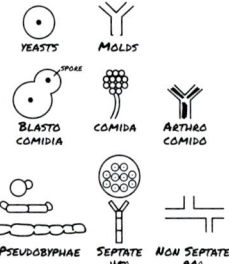

SKIN — ON SKIN: MALEZZIA FOLFUR, TINEA VERRICADOR, WOOD'S LAMP SPHAGETTI + MEATBALLS, SELENIUM SHAMPOO

IN SKIN: DERMATOPHUTES "TINEAS" CAPITES / COLPUS / PEDIS   ONUCHOMYCOSIS = ORAL

UNDER SKIN: SPOROTHRIX TOPICAL
(D) ROSE-GARDENERS → SOIL → LYMPHATICS → ASCENDS   POTASSIUM IODIDE
DAISY CHAIR CLUSTERS ↔ CIGAR-SHAPED YEASTS

DIMORPHOC SYSTEMIC		ENDEMIC	PHRARE	MICRO
	(D) HISTO	OHIO, MS. VALLEYS + CANADA + EAST COAST	FARMER FIELDS (CAVES)	INTRACELLULAR YEASTS, MACROPHAGES
PULMONARY	(D) BLASTO		WOODLANDS + STREAMS	BROCED BARED BUDDING YEASTS
ITRACONAZOLE	(D) COCCIDIO	SW US, MEXICO	ARID DESERTS	SPHERULES

OPPORTUNISTIC

CANDIDA ALBIGANS				FLUCONAZOLE
– ORAL	THRUSH		PSEUDOHYPHAE	
– VAGINAL	COTTAGE CHEESE		GEIM TUBER @37°C	
– ESOPHAGEAL	DYSPHAGIA			
– DISSEMINATED	TPN			
ASPERHILLUS				
– ABPA	"ASTHMA"		SEPTALE HYPHAE	VARICONAZOLES
– ASPERGILLOMA	CAVITARY LESIONS		45° ↓ DRACHES	
– ASPERGILLUS INVASIVE	HALO SIGN			
PCP	AIDS DNA, CD4 C200 INTERSTITIAL PNA		SILVER STAIN YEASTS	TMP-SMX
CRYPTOCOCAUS	AIDS MENINGITIS Seizures, 330 CMLT20		INDIA INK CRAG	AMPHoB + FLUCYTOSINE → FLUCONAZOLE
MUCOR	DNA, FACIAL SINUSES		NONSEPTATE HYPHAE >90°	AMPHoB

PLASMA MEMBRANE STRESS (ERGOSTEROL)

CELL WALL — 1,3B – GLUCAN / 1,6B – GLUCAN / CHITIN

PLASMA MEMBRANE — 1,3–B – GLUCAN SYNTHASE

POLYENES — PORE FORMERS

① POLYENES (ERGOSTEROL, 1,3B – GLUCAN)

④ ECHINOCANDINS

CELL WALL STRESS (1,3-B-GLUCAN)

ECHINOCANDINS
MICAFUNGIN — DISSEMINATED CANDIDA
CASPOFUNGIN — NEUTROPENIC FEVERS

AMPHOTERECIN B – ANY FUNGUS
– DISSEMINATED DIMORPHIC
– CRYPTOCOCCAL MENINGITIS
– MUCOR

NEPHROTOXIC – LIPOSOMAL
NYSTATIN
TOPICALLY – CANDIDA ALBICANS
SWISH + SPIT – ORAL CANDIDA
SWISH + SWALLOW – ESOPHAGEAL

② AZOLE — 14-OL DEMETHYLASE / LANOSTEROL

③ — SQUALENE EPOXIDASE
ALLYLAMINE
BENZYLAMINE

SQUALENE | GLUCAN

⑤ FLUCYTOSINE

DNA/ RNA METABOLITES
FLUCYTOSINE → 5-FU

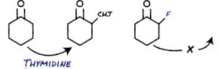

AMID AZOLES
KETON
ONICON — DERMATOPHYTE TOPICALLY
CLATRIM

ALLYLAMINE
TERBINAFINE
ONYOCHOMYCOSIS = PO

MITOTIC SPINDLE
⑥ GRISEOFULVIN

THYMIDINE SYNTHETASE
MITOTIC SPINDLE
~~ONYCHONYCOTIS~~

P-450-1
Triazoles — HEPATOXICITY
ANDROGEN-1 = GYNECOMASTIA

FLUZONAZOLE CANDILA ALBICANS INVASIVE ~~PISS~~

VORICONAZOLE ASPERGILLUS
ITRACONAZOLE DIMORPHIC INVASIVE ~~DISO~~

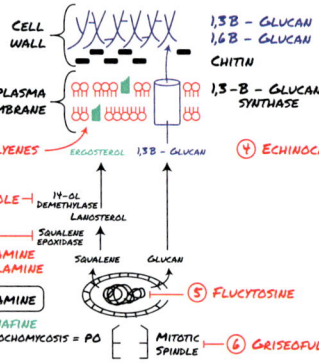

SIDE EFFECTS
EUCHARYOTIC — NUCLEUS, MITOCHONDRIA, 80N RIBOSOME
(P450)

NOTES

Protazoa

Intestinal

1. **E. Hystolitica (MTZ)**
   Bloody Diarrhea
   Flask-Shaped Ulcers, Colonic Mucosa
   Liver Abscesses, Anchovy Paste
   Trophozoite, 4 Nuclei, Ingested RBC

2. **Giardia Lamblia (MTZ)**
   Fatty Diarrhea = Steatorrhea
   Suction Cup, Prevents Absorption
   Pear-Shaped, Two Nuclei, Flagellated
   Camping/ Hiking

3. **Cryptosporidium**
   AIDS Diarrhea Watery Diarrhea
   Oocyst Acid-Fast Stain Stool

Urogenital

1. **Trichomonas (MTZ)**
   ∅ Cyst Form, P²P
   Flagellated, Motile, Wet Mount
   Vaginitis = Green Watery Discharge
   Ping-Ponging, Fx Both Partner

Malarial

1. **Malaria**
   Anopheles Mosquito, African
   Cyclical Fever + Anemia
   – Fevers = Merozoite – emia
   – Lysis = Anemia
   – Spleen = Anemia
   Plasmodium
   Malaria 72 Hrs
   Vivax
   Ovale } Hypnozoites
   Falciparum Fucks you up
   Ringed Trophozoites
   Schizont
   Mefloquine PPx/ Tx
   (Chloroquine Endomic Sens)

2. **Babesia = Malaria of US**
   Ixodes Tick (Lyme)
   Not-So-Cyclical, Undulating Fevers
   Lysis/ Spleen = Anemia
   Maltese Cross
   Atovaquone + Azithromycin

Other Ones

3. **Chagas Disease**
   T. Cruzi, Reduviid, South America
   Acute = CHF
   Chronic = Mega Colon, Mega Esophagus
   CHF Bxi Nonflag in Tissue

4. **African Sleeping Sickness**
   T. Brucei, Tsetse Fly, Africa
   Ulcer @ Bitesite
   Progressive Demyelinating
   Encephalitis

5. **Leishmania**
   L. Dionuami, Sandfly, Africa
   RES = HSM PLT↓
   Cutaneous

Brain

N. Fowleri
T. Gondii

Helmniths

Ascaris
A: Intestine, Steal Food
E: Stool, Contaminate Water, Ingestion ↑
L: Through GI to Lungs
   Malnutrition, Eggs, Stool

Ancylostoma
A: Intestine, Steals Blood
E: Stool, Hatch Soil
L: Through Skin to Lungs

Strongyloides
A: Intestine, Auto Infection
E: In Stool   In Colon
   Hatch   Hatch
L: Skin to Lungs GI to Lungs
   Gram⊕Bacteremia, Larvae

Enterobius NOT – Lung
A: Cecum, Deposits Perianal
E: Picked Up, Distributed
   Ingested ↑
L: Into   Not Through

Babies c̄ Itchy Butts
Adhesive Tape Test
Albendazole

Trichinella (DEH)
Encysted: Sk Muscle Pork/ Bear
Larvae
Encysted: Through GI to Sk Muscle
Larvae
Myositis, Muscle Weakness, ↑CPK

Toxocara Canis (DEH)
A: Dog Intestines
E: Food, Water
L: Through GI to Everywhere

S. Herub...

Schistosoma I   Bladder Cancer
A: Veins – Venous Plexus Bladder
   Urine
E: Water, Hatch Infect Snails,
   Free – Swimming
L: Skin to Home – Venous Plexus
   Squamous Cell Carcinoma

Schistosoma II   Cirrhosis
Water, Stool

Home = Mesenteric Veins
Granulomas/ Cirrhosis
↑Portel HTN

Taenia Neurocysticercosis
A:
E: Stool, Water, Humans
L: GI – Drain
   Albendazole + Steroids

Diphyllobothrium Fish, B12 Def
A: Intestine
E: Water, Eaten by Fish ↑ Raw
L: Fish Sk Muscle

Echinococcus (DEH)
A: Dog Intestine
E: Water/ Food, Ingested ↑
L: Through GI to Liver
   Hydatid Cystir
   Albendazole] Anaphylaxis

Clonorchis Cholangiocarcinoma
A: GB
E: Water, Stool
EL: Sk Muscle Fish

Tapeworm
Tapeworm
Stool, Water, Animal
GI – Muscle

NOTES